Miraculous Way of
Needles

OMAHHUM PUBLICATION

1st edition published by
©Omahhum Publication in 2016

Published by U.N. Acupuncture Center
307 E 44th Street, Suite B, NY, NY 10017, USA
medicalmidtown@gmail.com

Art and design by Dr. Tsoi Nam Chan
Calligraphy by Dr. Jiao Shun Fa

ISBN: 978-0-692-70016-7
Printed in New York, USA

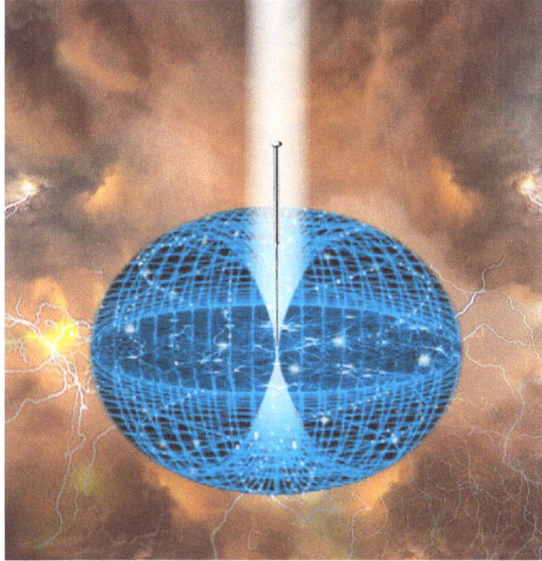

Miraculous Way of Needles

This pioneering work offers readers an entirely new interpretation of acupuncture's *Jingmai* theories, as postulated by Dr. Jiao Shun Fa. Dr. Jiao's work is based on ancient texts from the famous Chinese text, *The Yellow Emperor's Inner Canon*, as well as on 40 years experience developing clinical acupuncture treatments and conducting extensive medical research in the field of Chinese medicine. His medical writings include *Head Acupuncture, Jiao Shun Fa Head Acupuncture, Carotid Drip Liquid in the Treatment of Cerebrovascular Disease, Seeking the Truth of Chinese Acupuncture and Moxibustion, Soul of Chinese Acupuncture and Moxibustion, Acupuncture and Moxibustion Theory and Clinical Practice, Treating Diseases with Acupuncture* and more than ten other texts published in China and abroad. This new version of the classic Chinese medical text, the *Ling Shu - Nine Needles and Twelve Yuan-Source Points*, is his latest work and in many ways his most important contribution to the literature of contemporary Chinese medicine.

Acupuncture treatment is an ancient healing science developed by scholars millennia ago in ancient China. As early as 2500 B.C., its fundamental method of treating disease by inserting needles into key energy points throughout the body was explained in the first chapter of the *Ling Shu*. This groundbreaking book has remained a classic of Chinese medicine since the time it was written. Yet, due to misunderstandings of its sophisticated and complex content over the centuries, a substantial part of the *Ling Shu*'s essential teachings has been lost or misinterpreted. This loss, in turn, has had a profoundly negative impact on the transmission of accurate acupuncture knowledge, even up to the present day.

The time has come, therefore, for a new interpretation of this ancient text – an interpretation that revises the many errors and misinterpretations that have plagued this great work over the centuries, and that better captures its original meaning and intent. The present book, it is hoped, will provide this needed corrective, amending errors that have crept into the text, clarifying important medical issues, and presenting its luminous medical insights for the use of future generations to come.

Introduction

Dr. Jiao Shun Fa was born on December 25, 1938 in High Canal Village, Jishan County, West Commune in Shanxi province, China. He currently serves as professor and chief physician, where he is a member of the China Association of Acupuncture and Moxibustion, and Chairman of the Acupuncture and Moxibustion Society in Shanxi province.

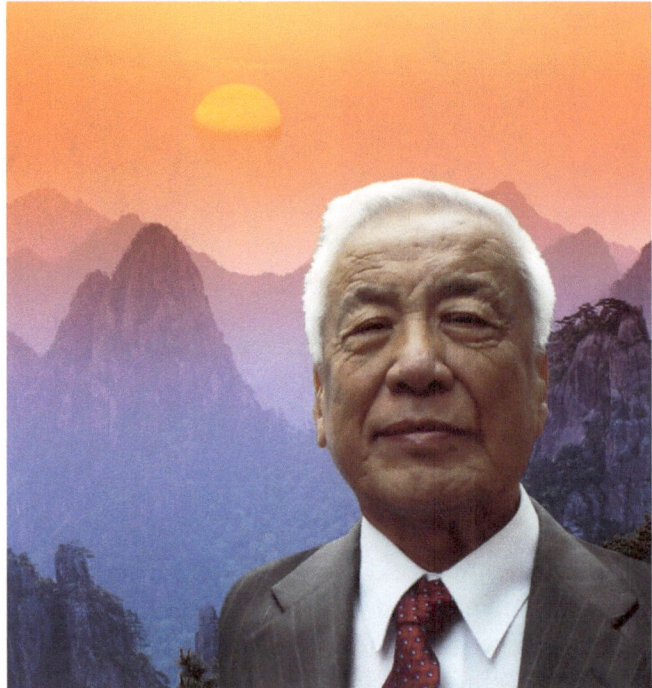

In 1970 Jiao Shun Fa invented "head acupuncture," a medical protocol that has been used successfully over the past several decades to treat a variety of brain disorders. In 1976, he developed a new treatment for cerebral vascular disease using carotid artery medicinal drips. Over the years, Dr. Jiao has promoted this method and its application throughout China. In 1986, he received a first prize National Award for his work in the field and for significant achievements in the development of Chinese medicine.

Dr. Jiao has worked tirelessly for more than 40 years developing clinical acupuncture treatments and conducting extensive medical research in the field of Chinese medicine. His medical writings include *Head Acupuncture, Jiao Shun Fa Head Acupuncture, Carotid Drip Liquid in the Treatment of Cerebrovascular Disease, Seeking the Truth of Chinese Acupuncture and Moxibustion, Soul of Chinese Acupuncture and Moxibustion, Acupuncture and Moxibustion Theory and Clinical Practice, Treating Diseases with Acupuncture*, and more than ten other texts published in China and abroad. His new version of the classic Chinese medical text, the *Ling Shu*, is his latest and in many ways most important contribution to the literature of contemporary Chinese medicine.

作者简况

　　焦顺发，1938年12月25日生于山西省稷山县西社乡高渠村。教授，主任医师。现任中国针灸学会常务理事，山西省针灸学会会长。

　　1970年发明"头针"，因对脑源性疾病有独特疗效，迅速在国内外应用。获1986年度国家中医药重大科研成果甲级奖。1976年发明了"颈动脉滴注药液治疗脑血管疾病"的新方法，并在全国推广应用。

　　40年来一直在针灸治病的临床和理论方面，进行广泛深入研究，并有独特见解。著有《头针》，《焦顺发头针》，《颈动脉滴注药液治疗脑血管疾病》，《中国针灸学求真》，《中国针灸魂》，《针灸原理与临床实践》，《针刺治病》等十余部专著，出版发行国内外。

Preface

Acupuncture treatment is an ancient healing science that was developed by scholars millenia ago in ancient China. As early as 2500 B.C., its fundamental method of treating disease by inserting needles into key energy points throughout the body was explained in the first chapter of the famous *Ling Shu - Nine Needles and Twelve Yuan-Source Points*. This groundbreaking book has remained a classic in Chinese medicine since the time it was written.

However, due to misunderstandings of its sophisticated and complex content over the centuries, a substantial part of the *Ling Shu's* essential teachings has been lost or misinterpreted. This loss, in turn, has had a profoundly negative impact on the transmission of accurate acupuncture knowledge, even up to the present day.

The time has come, therefore, for a new interpretation of this ancient text – an interpretation that revises the many errors and misinterpretations that have plagued this great work over the centuries, and that better captures its original meaning and intent.

The present book, it is hoped, will provide this needed corrective, amending errors that have crept into the text, clarifying important medical issues, and presenting its luminous medical insights for the use of future generations to come.

Jiao Shun-Fa
February 24, 2008

序

  针刺治病，起源中国，发展于中国。早在《灵枢·九针十二原第一》，即总结和倡导用微针刺经脉治病的绝妙方法，后因对原文破解有误，严重影响传承。因此，重新审视、正确解读、认真传承《九针十二原第一》价值非凡、意义重大。因其不仅能使中国古代医学家发明的，微针刺经脉治病方法，重见天日，大放异彩，而且还能继续引领中国针刺治病，再创辉煌。故成此书。

焦顺发
2008 年 2 月 24 日

Foreword

Though I have read *Nine Needles and Twelve Source Points* for more than 40 years, each time I delve into its profound writings I experience yet another new inspiration. One needs not only a calm mind and clear thoughts to read this text but also a capacity for bold decision making and a courageous initiative. Yet even now after all these years I make no claim to understanding this ancient text fully or to having plumbed its depths. At best I have formed a group of personal opinions about its teachings and have gained insights simply by being in daily contact with its wisdom. There is a saying in Chinese that speaks of "throwing bricks to attract jade." In other words, sometimes even an incomplete and imperfect attempt serves to help and motivate others. That is my intention with this present translation.

Jiao Shun-Fa
October 30, 2007

One needs not only a calm and clear mind to read *Nine Needles and Twelve Source Points* but also boldness in decision making and courage to take initiative.

Jiao Shun-Fa
February 27, 2007

Ling Shu Chapter 1- Nine Needles and Twelve Source Points sums up in depth research, core experiences and theoretical achievements of Chinese medical specialists in the treatment of disease with acupuncture over thousands of years. It advocates and promotes the treatment of disease by needling the *Jingmai*, and should be considered an advanced medical science for its rational theories, excellent methods, and unique therapeutic effects.

Jiao Shun-Fa
March 18, 2007

前記

  我读《九针十二原第一》已有 40 余载，每每读后都有新感受。但是到目前为止，还不敢说读懂，只能说在某些方面有自己的见解，或者说仅有点小得。尽管如此，我也愿意将其写出，抛砖引玉。敬请方家探讨和高人指点。

焦顺发
2007 年 10 月 30 日

  读《九针十二原第一》，需要冷静头脑，清晰思维，更需要大胆决策，勇敢创举。

焦顺发
2007 年 2 月 27 日

  《灵枢·九针十二原第一》，深入研究，认真总结了数千年以来，中国医学专家针刺治病的核心经验和理论研究成果。倡导和弘扬的针刺经脉治病是理论科学，方法绝妙，疗效独特的先进医学。

焦顺发
2007 年 3 月 18 日

"*DAO*"

Calligraphy by Dr. Jiao

©ZL 200930124815.0

Chapter 1 - Original Text - Summary of Notes
Section 1 - Summary of the Original Text

1 - Original Text: "The Yellow Emperor said to *Qi Bo*: I treat my people as if they were my own children. I feed them and collect land taxes from them. I have pity on their inability to take care of their own health and on their vulnerability to diseases. I want to protect them from being treated by (harsh) drugs or stone implements that may cause side effects and pain. To accomplish this feat I prefer to use fine needles that can be inserted into the skin. These needles activate the *Jingmai* (acupuncture meridians), regulate and nourish the *Qi* (life force) and blood, manage the currents and counter currents (of energy), and assemble the entering/exiting convergent points. This system of fine needle acupuncture can certainly be passed down to future generations and last forever. Still, it must adhere to a set of clear rules. It must be easy to use, difficult to forget, and become a classical doctrine. We must, therefore, summarize its teachings into chapters, clarify what is extrinsic in it and what is intrinsic, and define both an end and a beginning. In short, in order to make everything appear organized, we must create a book titled 'Acupuncture doctrine.' I would like to hear your opinion on this matter."

Summary of Notes: The Yellow Emperor explained to *Qi Bo* that people cannot afford the taxes they must pay due to illness. He wants to protect them from drug or stone implement treatment, and encourages the use of fine needles that pierce the *Jingmais* (that is, pierce the somatic nerves), thus regulating *Qi* and curing disease. [Please refer to Note 1 and 2 in Chapter 1, Section 1.2]

This method of treatment can definitely be transmitted to future generations, but legislation (organization) is necessary. You should, therefore, write a book termed "Acupuncture Doctrine." Divide this book into the following chapters: diagnosis of major illness, *Jingmai*, the distribution of nerves in the visceras and body surface, acupuncture methods, and principles of point selection. Write all this information down in true, simple language that makes the book easy to use and difficult to forget. This information will then be passed down from generation to generation, lasting for numberless years without cease. I would like to hear your views on this subject.

"JINGMAI"
Calligraphy by Dr. Jiao

第一章 – 原文白話摘要及札記

第一节 – 原文白話摘要

一、原文：黄帝问于岐伯曰：余子万民，养百姓而收其租税。余哀其不给，而属有疾病。余欲勿使被毒药，无用砭石，欲以微针通其经脉，调其血气，营其逆顺出入之会。令可传于后世，必明为之法。令终而不灭，久而不绝，易用难忘，为之经纪。异其章，别其表里，为之终始。令各有形，先立针经。愿闻其情。

白话摘要：黄帝对岐伯说，子民因疾病交不起租税，我想不用药物和砭石，仅用微针刺经脉（实为刺躯肢神经）[详见札记一、二]，通过调整治愈他们的疾病。

这种治病方法肯定能传于后世，但必须立法。应该写一本《针经》，分不同章节，主要把疾病的诊断，经脉——神经在内脏和体表的分布、针刺方法、选穴原则，写的真实简单，易用难忘。就可使其世代传承，久而不绝。我想听听你的看法。

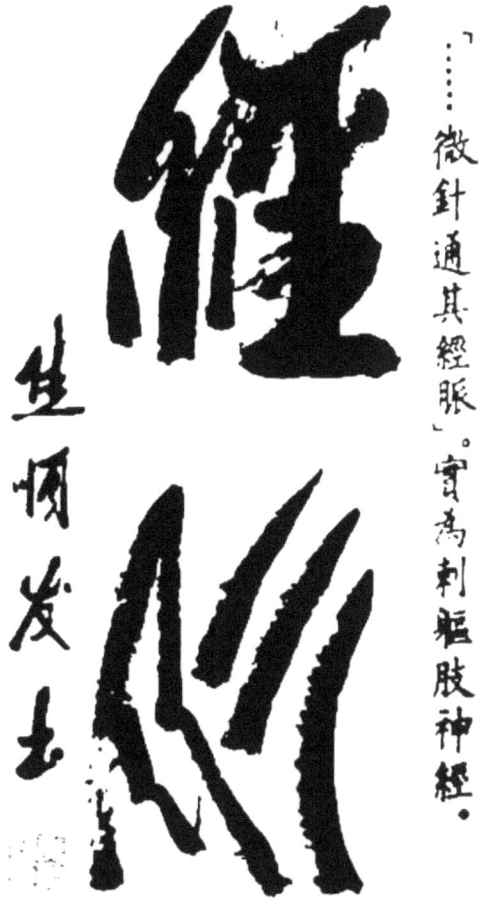

「……微针通其經脈」實為刺軀肢神經。

2 - Original Text: "A poor doctor knows only the physical location of an acupoint, while a superior doctor seeks the spirit (*Shen*) (inside the point). This spirit is wondrous; it is like a distinguished guest in the door."

Summary of Notes: An inferior doctor's only concern is which physical location on the body to perform acupuncture. A superior doctor knows how, when and where to needle the *Shen* point. *Shen* is very wondrous, like a distinguished guest in the door. *Shen* is described here. Refer specifically to the *Jingmai* within the acupoint - the body somatic nerves. Please refer to Note 3 in Chapter 1, Section 1.2.

T.N. Chan Interpretation: It could be that the needle is connected to the divine matrix.

"SHEN"
Calligraphy by Dr. Jiao

二、原文：粗守形，上守神。神乎神，客在门……

白话摘要：低劣的医生只知道针刺穴位，而高明的医生则知道在穴位中刺"神"。"神"非常神奇，就像尊贵的客人一样，分布在穴位之中。此处描述的"神"特指位于穴位中的经脉（躯肢神经）详见札记三。

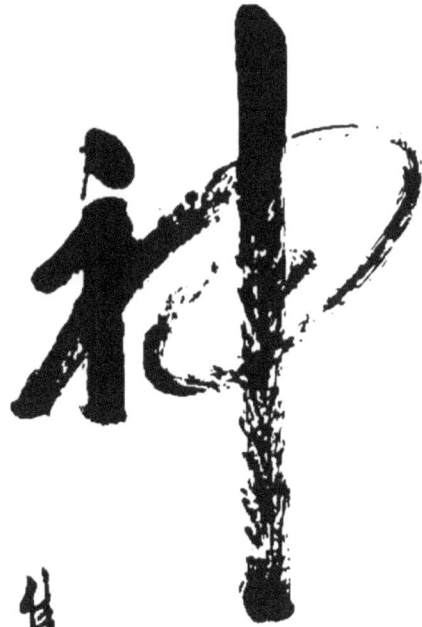

神

焦顺发

……"守神"特指守經脈，實爲刺躯肢神經。

©ZL 200930124819.9

3 - Original Text: "A poor doctor only knows how to look for the physical joints (*Guan*) while the superior doctor knows how to find *Ji* – gate mechanism in the point. The movement of *Ji* never exceeds its space. When we observe it from the outside *Ji* activity appears tranquil in the space it occupies. It appears to have only a slight movement. Its coming cannot be met and its going cannot be followed or grasped. Those who understand the gate mechanism are able to pierce the points precisely without missing a hair's breadth. Those who do not understand gate mechanism will miss the timing of *Qi*. Piercing points in a random way is useless. Knowing where *Qi* is coming from and where it is going and timing of *Qi* to get the best result is important. This phenomenon is really wondrous. The poor doctor remains in the dark (about it), while the superior doctor knows all these (important facts)."

Summary of Notes: Poor doctors only know how to perform acupuncture on the physical location of the points, while superior doctors know how to needle the gate, *Ji*. The *Ji* is located in the point itself, and its *Ji* activity at this point never exceeds its space. Through anatomical and physiological studies, they have found in the point of *Ji* that the surface appears outwardly tranquil with only slight pulsation. But in reality, information is being rapidly conveyed (in and out) of the *Ji*. Most doctors may not experience this fact through commonly used methods. By understanding the vital timing of the *Ji*, gate mechanism, it will be easy to pierce the target (reach the heart of the point). Not knowing the vital timing of the *Ji* mechanism is the same as locking the trigger (of a gun). Shooting will not be possible, and such random piercing is not going to hit the target. Poor doctors are in the dark about these principles, while superior doctors possess unique skills and can induce this wondrous phenomenon. Please refer to Note 4 in Chapter 1, Section 1.2.

"*JI*"
Calligraphy by Dr. Jiao

三、原文：粗守关，上守机。机之动，不离其空。空中之机，清静而微。其来不可逢，其往不可追。知机之道者，不可挂以发。不知机道，叩之不发。知其往来，要与之期。粗之暗乎，妙哉！工独有之。

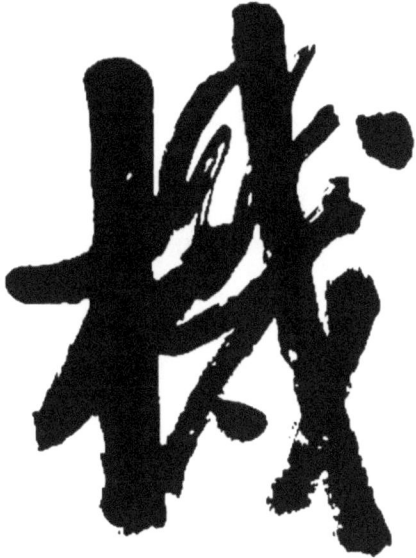

白话摘要：低劣的医生只知道针刺穴位，而高明的医生则知道在穴位中刺"机"。位于穴位中的"机"，活动范围从来不离开它的空间。经解剖，生理等研究发现位于穴位中的"机"，从表面看非常宁静，仅有微动。实际上其内部快速传递着出入往来的信息。一般人用普通的方法是无法感受的。知道"机"的要害，就容易刺中它。不知道其要害，乱刺是刺不中的。低劣的医生根本不知道这些，只有高明的医生才能领悟到其中的奥妙。详见札记四。

机

「……守機」。特指守經脈，實為刺軀肢神經。

焦顺发

©ZL 200930124818.4

4 - Original Text: "The term 'going' means 'counter flow.' The term 'coming' means to 'follow.' By knowing 'counter flow' and 'follow,' a doctor can perform acupuncture without asking (needless questions). *Qi* activity is not made deficient by withdrawing the needle with the tip going against the pathway of the *Jingmai*, and is not in excess by following the flow of the *Jingmai* with the needles. Counter flow and follow: if you understand this theory you definitely have mastered the great art of needling technique."

Summary of Notes: When applying acupuncture, the direction of needling that diminishes the "arrival of *Qi*" is described as "the direction of counter flow," while the direction that triggers the "arrival of *Qi*" is called "flow." By knowing the meaning of flow and counter flow you can insert the needle (without fear). Withdrawing the needle, the "arrival of *Qi*" will then be reduced; thrusting it during the "arrival of *Qi*" enhances it. Follow your instinct to regulate the intensity of *Qi* by moving the needle backwards and forward. This is the most important technique in clinical acupuncture.

5 - Original Text: "Deficiency by filling, excess by draining, chronic stagnation by eliminating, and over abundance of evil *Qi* by withdrawing."

Summary of Notes: For "deficiency by filling," one needs to needle the points repeatedly to promote *Qi* activity until signs of activity are obvious. This method is called "excess." Needling should stop when the *Jingmai* is activated. For "excess by draining" one should withdraw the needle a bit to relax the intensity of *Qi* activity. For "chronic stagnation by eliminating" the doctor must withdraw the needle slightly when it meets resistance and cannot be fully inserted, then change its direction. "Over abundance of evil *Qi* by withdrawing" refers to the process of pulling back the needle when there is obvious pain in order to stop unpleasant sensations. Please refer to Note 5 in Chapter 1, Section 1.2.

四、原文：往者为逆，来者为顺。明知逆顺，正行无问。迎（逆）而夺之，恶得无虚；追而济之，恶得无实；迎之随之，以意和之，针道毕矣。

白话摘要：在针刺的时候，能使气至消退的方向称"逆"，能使气至出现的方向称顺。知道逆顺之意，就大胆去刺，不要再问了。针迎而退，还能不使气至减弱，针推而进，还能不使气至增强。将针退或进，随意调整气至程度。这就是针刺的重要技术。

五、原文：虚则实之，满则泄之、宛陈则除之，邪胜则虚之。

白话摘要：虚则实之即是在针刺时，没有出现气至就反复刺，直到突然出现明显气至，即称"实"。表示已刺中经脉即立刻停止。满则泄之，则是出现气至太强烈，应将针往后退使其减弱一些。宛陈则除之，即是针遇到阻力刺不进去时，应将针往后推，改变方向再刺。邪胜则虚之，即是在针刺时，如果出现明显痛疼等异常感觉，应将针往后退，使其消失。详见札记五。

6 - Original Text: "*The Great Essentials* says: 'Slow, then rapid is excess. Rapid, then excess is deficiency. Speaking of excess and deficiency, sometimes it is there, sometimes it is not. As for examining before and after, sometimes it is there, sometimes it is not. Speaking of the feeling of empty and full, sometimes we gain it and sometimes we lose it.'"

Summary of Notes: This is an old text from ancient times. "Slow then rapid is excess" means that when the tip of the acupuncture needle reaches the correct depth of the *Jingmai*, push it in slowly. If *Qi* appears immediately, the needle tip is considered to be at the solids level. This "solidness" demonstrates that contact has been made with the *Jingmai* or somatic nerves. "Rapid then slow is empty" means that despite the fact that the piercing speed is fast and hard the *Qi* does not arrive. This means that the needle is still in the state of "emptiness" (that is, it has not yet pierced *Jingmai*), a condition that is referred to as "empty." Sometimes it is there, sometimes it is not." This phrase means that when needling *Jingmai* the solidness and emptiness that we talked about is sometimes there, while at other times it cannot be felt. When observing and comparing the situation before and after the arrival of *Qi*, sometimes there is sensation and sometimes there is no sensation. In reference to excess and deficiency, sometimes it is there, sometimes it is not there. That is to say, with emptiness and solidness, sometimes there is sensation and sometimes there is no sensation. Please refer to Note 6 in Chapter 1, Section 1.2.

7 - Original Text: "Needling precisely has to do with being quick and being slow."

Summary of Notes: Experienced doctors are able to contact the *Jingmai* (somatic nerves) and trigger the arrival of *Qi* very quickly. It is more difficult for poor doctors to pierce and hit the *Jingmai* in this way. The difference between the two is whether or not they can quickly trigger the arrival of *Qi*.

六、原文：《大要》曰："徐而疾则实，疾而徐则虚。言实与虚，若有若无；察后与先，若存若亡；为虚为实。若得若失。"

白话摘要：《大要》是上古时期的古经文。"徐而疾则实"即是针在穴位中，已接近刺中经脉的深度时，再将针徐徐往进推，如立刻出现明显的"气至"现象，表示针尖已到实处，简称"实"。实为刺中经脉（躯肢神经）。"疾而徐则虚"，即是如果进针速度较快，仍然没有出现明显气至现象，则表示针还在虚处，简称"虚"。证明没有刺中经脉（躯肢神经）。言实与虚，若得若失，即是在针刺经脉时。所说的实与虚，有时有，有时则没有感觉。察后与先，若存若亡，即是在先后对比观察，则有时有，有时则没有感觉。为虚为实，若得若失，即是所说的虚、实，有时有，有时则没有感觉。详见札记六。

七、原文：刺之微，在速迟。

白话摘要：有经验的医生容易刺中经脉（躯肢神经）。没有经验的医生刺中经脉（躯肢神经）比较困难，两者差别仅有快慢之分。

8 - Original Text: "To drain is called *Ying*. The meaning of *Ying* is to hold it inside, release and expel the Evil *Qi*, discharge *Yang*, and then remove the needle. Evil *Qi* can be drained in this way. To tonify is to follow. The sensation of following is as if to forget, to stimulate and press like a mosquito or gadfly bite, to detain and return, then to withdraw like an arrow leaving the bowstring. Command the left to follow the right; this will cause the *Qi* to stop."

Summary of Notes: Dispersion is called *Ying*. This means that to disperse you must have *Ying* energy present. The meaning of *Ying* is to push the needle into the acupoint and then insert it forward. When the sign of *Qi* arrival suddenly appears the patient often cannot stand the pain. At this point, you pull the needle backwards and the *Qi* arrival sensation will diminish or disappear.

To tonify is to follow. This means that to tonify one must push the needle into the acupoint. This specific technique calls for needling the acupoint, and piercing close to the *Jingmai* (somatic nerves) or when the tip of the needle is getting close to its surface. When the *Qi* has arrived, however, (the situation) is still not ideal and there is still need to tonify, to push the needle slowly inward. Be cautious here, stopping as soon as it is obvious that the *Qi* is reached. If the needle is pushed too quickly or forcefully, or if the direction is changed, the arrival of *Qi* may disappear entirely.

9 – Original Text: "As for the way to hold a needle, holding it tight is precious. Therefore, hold the needle straight and pierce perpendicularly. Do not needle to the left or right. Observe attentively. Watch the patient (carefully) while you work."

Summary of Notes: Hold the needle tightly and insert it perpendicularly. Observe closely. The arrival of *Qi Ji* proves that the needle has reached the *Jingmai* (the somatic nerve). At this point stop needling immediately.

"Tonify and Drain"
Calligraphy by Dr. Jiao

八、原文：泻曰迎之，迎之意，必持内之，放而出之，排阳得针，邪气得泄……补曰随之，随之意若妄（忘）之，若行若按，如蚊虻止，如留而（如）环，去如弦绝，令左属右，其气故止……

白话摘要：泻曰迎之，即是泻就说迎。迎的意思则是必须先将针在穴位中往进推，如突然出现明显气至现象，因程度严重，病人很难忍受时，则将针往后退，即可使过强的气至现象减弱或消失。

补曰随之，即补就叫往进推。具体推法是针在穴位中刺到接近经脉（躯肢神经），或已达其表面，气至现象出现的还不太理想，需要增补时，将针特别缓慢的往进推，边推边体验，一旦气至明显立刻停止。如果推的过快，或用力太大，或改变方向可使气至消失的一干二净。

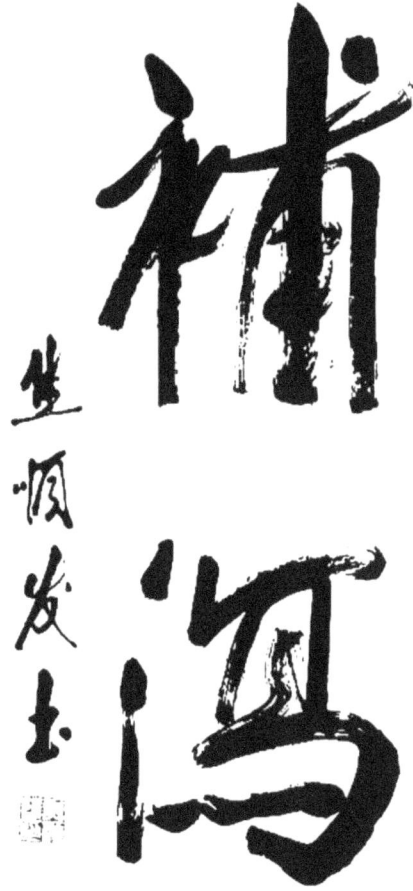

©ZL 200930124815.0

九、原文：持针之道，坚者为宝，正指直刺，无针左右；神在秋毫，属意病者……

白话摘要：捏紧针，垂直刺，认真观察，一旦出现明显气至，即证明已刺中经脉（躯肢神经），立刻停止。

10 - Original Text: "Piercing and *Qi* has not arrived. Don't ask how many times; pierce and *Qi* arrives, then remove the needle and no more piercing."

Summary of Notes: When using fine needles to pierce *Jingmai*, if there is no sign of *Qi Ji* appearing, do not worry about how many times you pierce. Simply continue piercing until *Qi Ji* arrives, then remove the needle and stop. Please refer to Note 7 in Chapter 1, Section 1.2.

11 - Original Text: "The essence of needling is that once *Qi* arrives a (healing) effect is generated. This effect appears quickly, as when the wind blows away the clouds, suddenly causing the sky to become clear and blue. This process describes the complete *Tao* of needling."

Summary of Notes: During acupuncture, as soon as *Qi* becomes active the therapeutic effect is obtained. This effect comes quickly, as when the wind suddenly blows away the dark clouds. Please refer to Note 8 in Chapter 1, Section 1.2.

十、原文：刺之而气不至，无问其数；刺之而气至，乃去之，无复针。

白话摘要：在用微针刺经脉时，如果无气至现象出现，不要管刺多少次，应反复刺，直到出现气至现象，就出针不要再刺了，详见札记七。

十一、原文：刺之要，气至而有效，效之信，若风之吹云，明乎若见苍天，刺之道毕矣。

白话摘要：在针刺的时候，一旦出现气至，就可获得确信的疗效。其效之快，如同风吹乌云散，详见札记八。

12 - Original Text: "The Yellow Emperor said, 'I would like to know about the origins of the five *Zang* and six *Fu* organs." *Qi Bo* replied, "Five *Zang*, Five *Shu*, five times five is 25 *Shu*. Six *Fu* and six *Shu*, six times six is 36 Shu. *Twelve Jingmai* and 15 *Luo Mai* constitute the 27 *Qi* pathways on which the *Qi* travels up and down. Where *Qi* comes out it is called *Jing* (the well) point, where it trickles it is called *Ying* (the spring) point, when it is poured it is called *Shu* (the stream) point. Where it runs it is called *Jing* (the river) point, and when it gathers it is called *He* (the lake) point. The 27 *Qi* pathways all depend on these five *Shu* points. Crossings of *Jie*, 365 junctions. For those who know the essence, one sentence is enough; those who do not know talk pointlessly and endlessly. The so-called *Jie* are places where *Shen Qi* travels in and out; they are not skin, muscles, tendons and bones.'"

Summary of Notes: The Yellow Emperor said he wished to know the origins of the five *Zang* and six *Fu* organs. *Qi Bo* said that the five *Zang* organs each have five *Shu* points. There is a total of 25 *Shu* points. Six *Zang* organs each have six Shu points making a total of 36 *Shu* points. There are 12 *Jingmai*, and 15 *Luo Mai*. The *Jing Qi* all have to go through the five *Shu* points.

In conclusion, he said "Crossings of *Jie*, 365 *hui*" means that the 365 points throughout the body are formed by junctions of *Jingmai* that cross each other many times. This knowledge is the result of scientific research done long ago. But (through the years) there have been different interpretations of this principle and experts have not been able to agree. So people say that "for those who know the essence, one sentence is enough; those who do not know talk pointlessly and endlessly." In modern times, the superior doctor summarizes the meaning of *Jie* in one statement, proclaiming that "*Jie* are junctions of the anterolateral and posterolateral spinal tracts and neurofilaments that cross multiple times. These junctions freely transmit (motional and sensory) information, and they are neither skin, muscles, tendons nor bones." Please refer to Note 9 in Chapter 1, Section 1.2.

"DU JIE"
Calligraphy by Dr. Jiao

十二、原文：黄帝曰：原闻五脏六腑所出之处。岐伯曰："五脏五腧，五五二十五腧；六腑六腧，六六三十六腧。经脉十二，络脉十五，凡二十七气以上下，所出为井、所溜为荥、所注为腧、所行为经、所入为合。二十七气所行，皆在五腧也。节之交，365会。知其要者，一言而终；不知其要，流散无穷。所言节者，神气之所游行出入也，非皮、肉、筋、骨也。"

白话摘要：黄帝说愿意知道五脏六腑所出之处。岐伯说，五脏各有五腧，五脏共有25腧。六腑各有六腧，六腑共有三十六腧。经脉十二，络脉十五，27条经脉之气的循行皆通过五腧穴。

最后他说，节之交，365会，即是全身的365个穴位都分布着由经脉之节多次交叉后形成的会。这是很久很久以前的科研成果。但后人破解不同，世代争论不息。所以有人感慨地说，"知其要者，一言而终；不知其要，流散无穷"。后来有高明的医生用一句话概括了"节"的含意。即所谓"节"者，（详见札记九）即是位于脊髓两侧的神经根（细）丝，因其通过多次交叉形成了躯肢神经，而且能自由传递出入（运动、感觉）信息，又不是皮、肉、筋、骨。详见札记九。

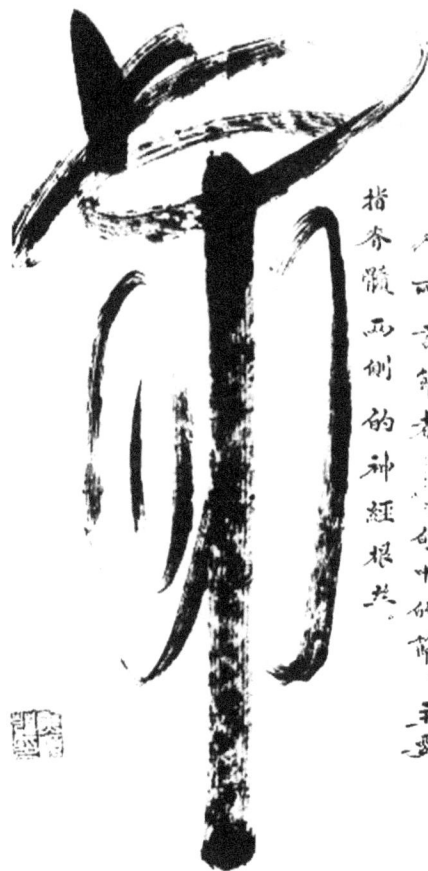

节

楷书髓而侧的神经根共

以四言节者之不句中的节，主要

13 - Original Text: "Observe the eyes; one can know (much from) their dilation and recovery."

Summary of Notes: By examining the size of the pupils, their shape, and their sensitivity to light, one can judge the condition of the patient. Please refer to Note 10 in Chapter 1, Section 1.2.

14 - Original Text: "Whenever one starts to practice acupuncture, one must check the patient's pulse, examine the condition of the patient's *Qi*, and then begin treatment."

Summary of Notes: Whenever doctors start to do acupuncture they must check the pulse to gauge the condition of the patient and confirm whether or not acupuncture is a suitable healing method for this particular disease.

15 - Original Text: "The five *Zang* and six *Fu* organs have 12 *Yuan*-source points. The 12 *Yuan*-source points originate from the four 'Guan' (elbow and knee joints). The four 'Guan' are used to treat diseases in the five *Zang* organs. When there is disease in the five *Zang* organs the 12 *Yuan*-source points should be chosen for treatment. The 12 *Yuan*-source points are the keys for the five *Zang* organs; (they help them) receive the *Qi* and the 'tastes' (essence) of the 365 *Jie* (points). When there is illness in one of the five *Zang* organs there will be reactions appearing in the 12 *Yuan* (source) points. The 12 source points have their outlet points (for these reactions) respectively. Knowing their source clearly and seeing their reactions, the doctor can identify disease in the five *Zang* organs. For the lung, the *Yuan*-source point is originated from LU 9 (*tài yuān*). For the heart, the *Yuan* point is from PC 7 (*dà lín*). That of liver is at LV 3 (*tài chōng*). That of spleen is at SP 3 (*tài bái*). That of kidney is at KI 3 (*tài xī*). That of *Gao* is at RN 15 (*jiū wěi*), and that of the *Huang* is at RN 6 (*qì hǎi*). All of these 12 source points (are used to) treat the diseases of the five *Zang* and the six *Fu* organs of the body."

十三、原文：察其目，知其散复……

白话摘要：观看瞳孔的大小，形状和对光反应的灵敏度判断病情。详见札记十。

十四、原文：凡将用针，必先诊脉，视气之剧易，乃可以治也……

白话摘要：凡是用针刺经脉治病者，必须先切脉诊断病情，确定能否针刺治疗。

十五、原文：五脏有六腑，六腑有十二原。十二原出于四关，四关主治五脏。五脏有疾，当取之十二原，十二原者，五脏之所以禀三百六十五节气味也。五脏有疾也，应出十二原。十二原各有所出，明知其原，睹其应，而知五脏之害矣。……肺也，其原出于太渊，太渊二。……心也，其原出于大陵，大陵二。……肝也，其原出于太冲，太冲二。……脾也，其原出于太白，太白二。……肾也，其原出于太溪，太溪二。膏之原，出于鸠尾，鸠尾一。肓之原穴出于脖胦（气海）。凡此十二原者，主治五脏六腑之有疾者也。

Summary of Notes: There are five *Zang* and six *Fu* organs. The six *Fu* have 12 source points. Although those 12 source points are located at the end of the body's four limbs, they are nonetheless connected to the five *Zang* and six *Fu*. Therefore, when there is disease in the *Zang* and *Fu* organs, the 12 source points should be chosen for treatment. These 12 source points have their origins respectively. The *Yuan*-source point of the lung is originated from from LU 9 (*tài yuān*), that of heart is from PC 7 (*dà líng*), that of liver is from LV 3 (*tài chōng*)... that of spleen is from SP 3 (*tài bái*), that of kidney is from KI 3 (*tài xī*), that of the *Gao* is from RN 15 (*jiū wěi*), and that of the *Huang* is from RN 6 (*qì hǎi*). All of these 12 source points are used treat the disease of the five *Zang* and the six *Fu* organs.

16 - Original Text: "Diseases of the five *Zang* organs are like thorns, dirty stains, knotted ropes or (dense) obstructions. (Yet), even thorns that nestle in the flesh for a long period of time can be pulled out. Even old stains can be cleaned. Even knots can be untied and obstructions cleared. It is wrong to believe that chronic diseases can never be cured. Those who are skillful at acupuncture can remove disease as if they were pulling out a thorn, cleaning a stain, opening a knot or clearing up blockages. Chronic diseases can be put to an end. People who say chronic diseases are incurable have not fully mastered the technique of using fine needles to pierce the *Jingmai*."

Summary of Notes: (Chronic) disease in the five *Zang* is like a thorn, a knot, or a flowing river that is partially or fully blocked. Even though a thorn has been in the skin for a long period of time, however, it can still be pulled out, just as old stains can be washed away, knots that have been tied for a long time can be loosened, and rivers that have long been blocked can be cleared. Some people say chronic disease cannot be cured. This notion is incorrect. The technique of using fine needles to pierce *Jingmai* (somatic nerves) can be used to treat chronic diseases just as a thorn can be pulled from the skin, a stain can be cleaned, and the blockades in a river removed. People who say chronic diseases are incurable have not fully mastered the technique of using fine needles to pierce *Jingmai* (somatic nerves).

白话摘要：五脏有六腑。六腑有十二原穴。十二原穴虽然位于四肢末端，但其通五脏六腑，所以脏腑之疾病当取十二原穴治疗。原穴各有所出，肺的原穴出于太渊（2），心的原穴出于大陵（2），肝之原穴出于太冲（2），脾之原穴出于太白（2），肾之原穴出于太溪（2），膏之原穴出于鸠尾，肓之原穴出于脖胦脖（气海）。此十二原穴治疗五脏六腑之疾病。

十六、原文：今夫五脏之有疾也，譬犹刺也，犹污也，犹结也，犹闭也。刺虽久，犹可拔也；污虽久，犹可雪也；结虽久，犹可解也；闭虽久，犹可决也。或言久疾之不可取者，非其说也。夫善用针者，取其疾也，犹拔刺也，犹雪污也，犹解结也，犹决闭也。疾虽久，犹可毕也。言不可治者，未得其术也。

白话摘要：五脏有病，就像扎了刺，有了污点，绳子打了结，河道堵塞一样。但是刺虽扎的久，仍可拔掉。污虽久，仍可洗掉。结虽久，仍可解开，河道堵塞，仍可疏通。有人说病久了不能治，这种说法是错误的。用微针刺经脉（躯肢神经）的方法，就像拔刺，洗污，解结，清堵一样将其治愈。说久病不能治者，是其没有掌握了微针刺经脉（躯肢神经）的技术。

Section II notes

I. Reflections on the first paragraph of *Ling Shu Chapter 1 – Nine Needles and Twelve Source Points*.

In *Ling Shu Chapter 1 - Nine Needles and Twelve Source Points*, the Yellow Emperor says to *Qi Bo*, "I treat my people as if they were my children, feed them and collect land taxes from them. I have pity on their inability to take care of their own health and their vulnerability to diseases. I want to protect them from (harsh or useless) treatment by means of drugs or stone implements which may bring about side effects and pain. I prefer to use fine needles that can be inserted into the skin to activate the *Jingmai* and regulate and nourish *Qi* and blood, and manage the junctions where *Qi* flow and counter flow exit and enter. The art of using fine needle acupuncture treatment can certainly be passed down to the future generations. It must be easy to use, difficult to forget, and (ultimately) become a classical doctrine. Summarize this information into chapters. Clarify the extrinsic and the intrinsic. Define an end and a beginning. In order to make everything appear organized, we should start to write a book called 'Acupuncture doctrine.' I would like to hear your opinion."

Medical scholars have attempted to interpret and apply this paragraph ever since it was first written. Most have come up with oversimplified interpretations, missed the mark concerning the passage's deep importance, and failed to demonstrate its true and original meaning. For the fact is that this paragraph is the single *most important passage* in the entire *Ling Shu*. Why? Because it explicitly defines the stimulation of the *Jingmai* with fine needles as the most scientific and effective method there is for treating disease. The author of *Ling Shu* hoped that this system would last a long time and be widely applied by later generations to come.

This opening paragraph is thus not only marvelous and unique, but is highly sophisticated and thoroughly scientific. It should be regarded as the main principle of the *Ling Shu* and viewed as the core and soul of all acupuncture practice and theory. In short, this passage describes thoroughly and superbly the treatment of disease by needling the *Jingmais*. It succinctly cuts through all mystery (and obscurity), leaving informed readers in awe.

第二节 - 札記

一、读《九针十二原第一》首段之悟

《灵枢·九针十二原第一》曰："黄帝问于岐伯曰：余子万民，养百姓，而收其租税。余哀其不给，而属有疾病。余欲勿使被毒药，无用砭石，欲以微针通其经脉，调其血气，营其逆顺出入之会，令可传于后世，必明为之法。令终而不灭，久而不绝，易用难忘，为之经纪。异其章，别其表里，为之终始。令各有形。先立《针经》。愿闻其情。"

该段经文闻世后，历代医家诠释，承用。但多据文字简单破解，一般处理，由此使其没有显露出原貌，更没有发挥其应有的作用。其实，该段经文是《灵枢》中最特别的一段。在独特的位置，描述最核心的问题，最有价值。因其将中国几千年的针刺治病，彻底进行了一次大清理，大总结；也是一次大飞跃、大变革。其明确表示用微针刺经脉是最科学、最有效的治病方法，作为成熟技术，期盼广泛应用，期待世代传承。

该段经文奇妙而特别，精炼而科学，应视其为《灵枢》的总纲、导读……为中国针刺治病的核心、灵魂……总之，该段经文将中国针刺经脉治病描述的淋漓尽致，出神入化，也可以说是一语道破天机，令人震憾！

"I prefer to use fine needles that can be inserted into the skin to activate *Jingmai* and regulate and nourish *Qi* and blood, manage the junctions where *Qi* flow and counter flow, exit and enter." This sentence should be considered the core message of this first paragraph.

Approximately 5,000 years ago, Chinese medical experts began to explore methods of needling the trunk and extremities in order to treat disease. In these early days doctors used thick needles to penetrate tissue and even the vital organs. They found that by needling the trunk and extremities they could sometimes bring about healing, an effect that was likely related to the fact that their needles occasionally (and accidentaly) stimulated the *Jingmai*. This random method, however, frequently caused serious injury to patients and even death. The *Treatise on Needling Contraindications* was thus intentionally included in *Huang Di Nei Jing-Su Wen* to warn doctors against needing important organs and tissues, and to urge them to use fine rather than thick needles in their clincal practice.

Using fine needles to activate the *Jingmai* is a wonderful and unique method for treating disease. The idea that doctors should use such needles in acupuncture was an innovation, a kind of technological revolution. Fine needles themselves are very mysterious. *Nine Needles and Twelve Source Points* describes the point of the fine needle as being similar to the stinger of a mosquito. It also describes the tip of a fine needle as being extremely thin, almost too small to be seen with the naked eye. Millennia ago, when people first started practicing acupuncture, they used thick needles in various shapes and sizes, some quite large and ungainly. Through years of clinical practice the advantages and disadvantages of different needles were tested, and fine needles eventually emerged as the safest and most efficient tool. Although there were several good reasons for using fine needles, the primary benefit was that they could easily puncture the skin and stimulate the *Qi*, leading to a favorable therapeutic effect free from side effects. The doctors of the time settled on fine needles as an optimal tool to activate the *Jingmai*, and as the most effective and scientific method for treating disease.

"欲以微针通其经脉，调其血气，营其逆顺出入之会。"应视为核心内容。因在当时针具繁多，方法杂乱，理解各异，在此时特别提出"微针通其经脉，调其血气，营其逆顺出入之会"，绝对不是描述过去所有的针刺治病技术，而是对中国几千年前，运用不同针刺各组织治病的大总结。

因大约在 5000 年前，中国医学专家就开始探索，针刺躯肢治疗病证的方法。初开始，运用针刺躯肢，并不完全都是刺经脉，而是不同组织都被刺中过，其中还刺中过重要脏腑和组织，并引起严重损害，甚至死亡。所以，在《黄帝内经·素问》中特编排了《刺禁论篇》告诫同仁，千万再不要刺中重要脏腑和组织。因在那个时段，用针在躯肢刺入其它组织，有时也会出现一些疗效（这可能与刺中这些组织中的经脉有关）。

用微针通经脉，奇妙而独特。微针本身即神秘莫测。微针包含毫针，《九针十二原第一》曰："毫针者，尖如蚊虻喙……经文描述的毫针尖部非常细，在当时这是人类肉眼看见的比较细小的物体。为什么要用这么细的针呢？这也正是奥妙奇特之处。此时提出用微针，即是针具的特殊革新，也是一场技术革命。因在很久以前，开始针刺经脉时，用的针比较粗，可能还有不同形状。后经长时间临床实践，一再证实不同针的优缺点，最后才确定为微针（包括毫针）。择用微针，虽原因诸多，但其中主要是易刺中经脉出现"气至"现象，获得较好疗效，又无明显损害（副作用）。所以，用微针通其经脉，是中国医学专家最后选择出针刺经脉的最佳针种（型），和最有效、最科学的针刺治病方法。

The statement that needling "regulates *Qi* and blood" should be viewed as a significant discovery. "Regulate" refers to the regulatory functions that needles provide when needling the *Jingmais*. These functions include changes in the blood supply and increased *Qi* flow into the affected areas. This discovery not only revealed the principle behind treating disease but also showed that the body's *Jingmai* system exerts a powerful regulatory function on the whole body. Thus, people can maintain health by regulating their *Jingmai* systems and achieving a balance between the interior and exterior parts of the body. If the body is attacked by a disease, the disease can be completely cured by proper needling of the respective *Jingmai*.

"Manage its junction of flow and counter flow and entering/exiting points" is another profound scientific observation. *Ying* refers to managing the substances that nourish the body, as well as the *Jingamis* related to disease. Here, "*Shun ni chu ru zhi hui*" particularly refers to the somatic *Jingmais*. In terms of function they deliver information in and out; in terms of structure they cross many times, forming junction points.

As a result, it is known that the method of using fine needles to pierce *Jingmais* provides a scientific healing method that is mature and technologically advanced, a method that can be promoted and applied to resolve the health care problem of the people of China.

When we witness the discoveries that the ancients made 1800 years ago in the fields of neurology and physiology we learn that the *Jingmai* they identified were actually what modern science knows today as the somatic nerves. This means that as early as 2,500 years ago, when most of the world's medical knowledge was at a Stone Age level, Chinese medical experts were intimately familiar with the human nervous system, and were treating disease with a highly sophisticated system of needle stimulatiion and *Qi*/blood regulation.

"Can be pased down to the future generations" and "lasts forever." These definitive sentences tell us that the art of using fine needles to pierce the *Jingmai* is so effective that its techniques will be passed down from generation to generation, a prediction that has allready proven true many times over. Today, as a doctor who uses fine needles to treat disease in my own practice, I feel great warmth and excitement by reading these beautiful predictive sentences written 1800 years ago.

"调其血气"应视为重大发现。"调"即调解也。指针刺经脉后，由于调解作用，使病损部位血液供应和气（某些功能）发生改变。这一发现，不仅揭示了针刺经脉治病的原理，而且证明了人体的经脉系统为调解系统（有很强的调解功能）。说明人体在平常通过经脉系统调解，达到体内，外平衡，保持健康。而在某些病损后，通过针刺相关的经脉进行调解，使病损痊愈。

　　"营其逆顺出入之会。"是一项重大科研成果。因"营"指营养。"其逆顺出入之会"，特指病损相关的躯体经脉。在此刻意用"逆顺出入之会"表述人体的躯肢经脉，即表示在功能上可传递逆顺出入之信息，在结构上交叉后能形成会。

　　由此而知，此处将微针刺经脉治病的方法，当成科学的治病方法，先进的成熟技术，广泛推广应用，解决中国民众的医疗保健。

　　时隔 1800 年后，用已知的神经解剖，生理等知识，进行对比研究发现，中国古代医学家发现的经脉、针刺治病的经脉，就是人体的躯体神经。据此证明，早在 2500 年前，在世界医学对人体神经系统认知甚少，茫然无知之时，中国医学专家就发现和深入研究了人体的神经系统。开创了用微针刺躯体神经，通过调解血气使功能改变，达到治病目的。这是中国医学的伟大发现和重大科研成果。

　　"令可传于后世……""令终而不灭，久而不绝……"这些绝句，明确告知，用微针刺经脉的治病方法，肯定能传于后世，而且可世代相传，久传不绝。时隔 1800 年后的今天，身为继续运用毫针刺经脉治病的临床实践家，亲眼目睹这些佳句，亲口读出这些经文，颇感亲切，兴奋无比。为此，我们一定要正确对待，认真传承。

II. Reflections on "… I prefer to use fine needles to open up its *Jingmai*, to regulate its *Qi* and blood, and to manage its junctions where *Qi* flow and counter flow, exit and enter. To pass it down to future generations, it is necessary to set clear rules."

"I prefer to use fine needles to open up its *Jingmai*, to regulate its *Qi* and blood, and to manage its junctions where *Qi* flow and counter flow, exit and enter. To pass it down to future generations, it is necessary to set clear rules."

This passage, taken from the first paragraph of *Ling Shu - Nine Needles and Twelve Source Points* develops a master principle of Chinese medicine, and presents us with a very important and unusual concept indeed. At the time of its writing many Chinese physicians did not have a clear understanding of its meaning, and over the centuries this led to many difficulties and misunderstandings. As I reread these cogent and ground-breaking sentences today I feel a heartfelt surprise. The following are my thoughts on these writings. Feedback and advice on these thoughts from experts would be appreciated.

(A) Interpretation by most Chinese physicians:

Over the centuries many medical specialists attempted to interpret the content of the *Ling Shu* by explaining it in superficial ways and developing contradictory versions of its teachings. This is why people of subsequent generations slowly lost interest in the text, and why there is something of a prejudice against it even today among modern practitioners. Up until the present era the *Ling Shu* continues to remain misunderstood, unstudied, and ignored.

(B) My specific interpretations according to the doctrines:

a. "Thus, I prefer to use fine needles to open up the *Jingmai*" is a technical phrase concerning the treatment of disease. It refers to the art of using fine needles to pierce *Jingmai* and hence unblock *Jingmai Qi*. This quote effectively summarizes treatment methods used 2,500 years ago up till today.

b. Chinese medical experts have not reached a consensus on the ultimate meaning of *Jingmai*. There are various reasons for this lack of consensus, first among them being resistance to taking seriously the all important sentence: "wishing to use fine needles to activate *Jingmai*."

二、读"……欲以微针通其经脉，调其血气，营其逆顺出入之会。令可传于后世，必明为之法。"之感悟

"……欲以微针通其经脉，调其血气，营其逆顺出入之会。令可传于后世，必明为之法。"

位于《灵枢·九针十二原第一》的首段中，是撰写《灵枢》的总纲，重要而特殊。然而，由于医学家们，对其破解有误，处理不当，致使后人对其理解、承用困难。笔者近期重读该段经文，心灵再次受到强烈震憾。现摘述于后，呈方家探讨和高人指点。

（一）一般人的诠释

《灵枢》闻世后，曾有很多专家对其进行过诠释。但是，多据字面含意进行简单破解。如"用微针疏通经脉（有些是刺肌肤），调理血气，增加经脉气血的逆顺出入来治疗疾病。要想使这种方法世代相传，必须明确提出针刺大法……"不同版本，大同小异。此类诠释和处理，致使后人对其淡化、偏见。也由此使其在《灵枢》中，一直尘封到今天。

（二）我据经文具体破解

1. 、"欲以微针通其经脉"，是中国古代针刺经脉治病中常用的一个专业术语。它既代表用毫针刺经脉，又有经脉被刺后能使经脉之气通达之意。该句经文是认真总结了前 2500 年，用不同针在躯肢各种组织针刺治病的方法和经验，结合其它科研成果特意写的。然而，在 2000 年后的今天。

2. 、中国医学专家，对针刺经脉的认识，仍然达不成共识。形成此种局面，虽有诸多原因，其中没有读懂或没有认真对待"欲以微针通其经脉"，即是主要原因之一。

1. "*Tiao Qi Qi Xue*" - "Regulating *Qi* and blood"

The term "Regulating *Qi* and blood," represents a significant scientific breakthrough, especially as it relates to the use of acupuncture and *Jingmai* for treating disease. While scholars have agreed on this point, the key mechanism of the phrase has only been passed down through the years by oral transmission, since memorization and repetition are more common than intensive research.

2. "Manage its junctions where *Qi* flow and counter flow, exit and enter."

When deciphering the phrase "manage the junctions where *Qi* flows and counter flows, exit and enter" one should first understand the meaning of the abstruce term "junctions where *Qi* flows and counter flows, exit and enter." One should also understand why we use this term. When I first started to read this phrase almost 40 years ago I was completely lost. Years later I finally discovered that "junctions where *Qi* flow and counter flow, exit and enter" was by no means a casual description but was based on experience with anatomy, physiology and other scientific research, combined with deep thought and inspired deliberation.

Ling Shu includes separate chapters on the 12 *Jingmai*, the 12 *Jing Bie* (divergent *Jingmai*), and the 12 *Jin Jing* (the tendons and the muscular system that run along the *Jingmai*). Yet the authors of the *Nine Needles and Twelve Source Points* did not use the information from these chapters to describe the *Jingmai*. Why? Because they disagreed with the notion that the *Qi* of the 12 *Jingmai* travels in one direction. And so, based on conclusions reached from their own scientific research, they created the entirely new expression, "Junctions where *Qi* flows and counter flows, exits and enters" to describe the *Jingmai* as they understood it.

2、"调其血气"

"调其血气"也是中国古代针刺经脉治病中常用的一个专业术语。它是对针刺经脉治病理论研究的重大科研成果。后来，业内人士一直认同此种说法。但是，单纯承述多，具体研究少。由此使"调其血气"的重要治病机理，一直仅流传于口头。

3、"营其逆顺出入之会"

破解"营其逆顺出入之会"，首先应知道，什么是"逆顺出入之会"？为什么要用"逆顺出入之会"？说实话，"逆顺出入之会"确实难懂。我在 40 年前开始读"逆顺出入之会"时，就根本不知道是什么意思。多年后才发现"逆顺出入之会"，不是随便写的，而是根据解剖、生理等多项科研成果，经过深思熟虑后，刻意这样写的。

因《灵枢》中不仅收录了十二经脉、十二经别、十二经筋……而且各自独立成篇。由此而知，《九针十二原第一》的作者，没有使用这类内容表述经脉，不是他们不懂或者写错了，而是不同意其中描述的十二经气单方向循行等内容，根据他们自己的科研成果，另辟蹊径，独创"逆顺出入之会"，表述躯肢经脉的方法。为什么这样说呢？

"Crossings of *Jie*, 365 junctions. For those who know the essence, one sentence is enough; those who do not know talk pointlessly and endlessly. The so-called '*Jie*' are places where *Shen Qi* travels in and out; they are not skin, muscles, tendons and bones."

I discovered that the above passage has a special relationship with the phrase "the junctions of counter flow, flow, exiting and entering points." In other words, we can say that "the junction of counterflow, flow, exiting and entering points" is a reference to "Crossings of *Jie*, 365 junctions," and that "the so-called '*Jie*'" refers to where the *Shen Qi* (spirit energy) travels in and out.

Here it is necessary to be specific in clarifying the term "Crossings of *Jie*, 365 junctions." This sentence, we know, existed before the publication of *Ling Shu* (though the actual date of its writing cannot be verified). It was, however, clearly based on important findings made by ancient Chinese doctors during their anatomical researches on *Jingmai*. From an early date it was then applied in disease treatment by using fine needles to pierce *Jingmai*. Unfortunately, because this finding was so ancient, later medical experts did not comprehend its real meaning and many misinterpretations occurred.

"Those who do not understand the essence talk pointlessly and endlessly." This phrase refers to the above mentioned tendency towards misinterpretation. "For those who know the essence, one sentence is enough." That is to say, for those who know the real meaning of *Jie*, one sentence is enough. "The so-called *Jie* are places where *Shen Qi* travels in and out, they are neither skin, muscles, tendons nor bones" expresses the meaning of *Jie* in one pithy sentence.

因为我读本篇的"节之交，365 会。知其要者，一言而终；不知其要，流散无穷。所言节者，神气之所游行出入也，非皮，肉，筋，骨也。"

之后，发现这段经文与"逆顺出入之会"有特殊关系。也可以说，"逆顺出入之会"，就是"节之交，365 会"；"所言节者，神气之所游行出入也"的缩写。

在这里要特别说明一下，"节之交，365 会"在《灵枢》成书前早就形成了（形成的确切年代现无据可查）。它是中国古代医学专家，经过解剖等对经脉实质研究的重大科研成果，并在针刺经脉治病中广泛应用。遗憾的是因其形成的年代太久远，后代医学专家因不解其意，出现过多种错误的诠释。

"不知其要，流散无穷"，就是上述状况的真实写照。知其要者，一言而终"。即是说知道"节"的真实含意者，一句话就说清楚了。"所言节者，神气之所游行出入也，非皮，肉，筋，骨也"。即是用一句话说清了"节"的含意（概况）。

By the time *Ling Shu* was published Chinese medical experts had developed the deepest and the most authoritative interpretation of *Jie* and "Crossings of *Jie*, 365 junctions." Here the author presented his conclusions based on his anatomical, physiological, and pathological studies, and then abstained from referring to other medical principles and issues.

However, after my in-depth study of the expert's summary of the special function of *Jie* and its scope, I found that the *Jie* is *not* a joint in the anatomical sense, nor is it the junction of joints. A joint in the anatomical sense cannot be the place where *Shen Qi* (spirit energy) travels in and out. Rather, it belongs to the category of bone structure. The true meaning of *Jie*, therefore, refers to the anterolateral and posterolateral spinal tracts and neurofilments, which are the pathways for the outgoing impulses of nerve motion and the incoming sensory information. They are not, as is sometimes believed, skin, muscles, tendons, and bones.

Based on this view we know that the phrase "Junctions where *Qi* flows and counter flows, exits and enters" refers to the somatic nerves that are formed by crossing spinal nerves. This term thus offers a simple and accurate expression of *Jingmai* in the human body, revealing the true meaning of the term "*Shen Qi* (spirit energy) travels in and out." Unfortunately, most medical experts have not understood its true meaning, and it is heartbreaking to see how their misconceptions have so negatively affected the inheritance and development of Chinese acupuncture.

这是在《灵枢》成书时，中国医学专家，对"节之交，365 会"中的"节"，理解最深，最权威的破解和表述。在此，他只讲了通过解剖，生理，病理等研究的结论性意见，没有讲其它。我根据专家对"节"概括的特殊功能及界定范围，

深入研究后发现，"节"根本不是指关节、关节相交处。因此处既不能使神气游行出入，又属骨的范畴；而是指脊髓前外侧沟的神经根（细）丝和后外侧沟的神经根（细）丝。因其通过脊髓能自由地传出运动冲动和传入感觉信息，又不是皮，肉，筋，骨。

由此而知，"逆顺出入之会"当然是指脊神经交叉后形成的躯肢神经。所以，用"逆顺出入之会"表述躯肢经脉，不仅简明扼要，而且又能表达其能使"神气之所游行出入也"的真实含意。遗憾的是，由于医学家们始终没有读懂"逆顺出入之会"，逼使中国针刺经脉治病，沿着破解之意不断变异，严重影响了对其的继承和发展，令人揪心。

4. The Three "*Qi*" ("its")

"*Qi*" is a pronoun meaning either "it, them, its" or "that, those." For the sake of brevity, this paragraph uses three "its" to refer to the body part that contains a disease.

For example "Use fine needles to open up its *Jingmai*" *means* to pierce the *Jingmai* associated with a disease using fine needles. "Regulate its *Qi* and blood" means to regulate the *Qi* and blood of the body part that contains the disease. "Managing its junction where *Qi* flows and counters flow, exits and enters" means to manage the *Jingmai* that control or are associated with the disease.

In light of this context, to apply acupuncture to the *Jingmai* does not mean that the doctor randomly pierces points over the entire body. Instead, acupuncturists must first identify the location of the disease and then pierce the specific *Jingmai* that control or are associated with the disease. By so doing they regulate the *Qi* and blood of the body part that contains the disease, enhance the function of the *Jingmai* associated with this disorder, and thus cure the disease. Unfortunately, previous interpretations failed to take into account the proper use of the term "its." As a result, the meaning of the text was distorted, making it difficult to understand, and even more difficult for future generations to apply.

5. "Passed it on to the future generations, it is necessary to make clear rules."

"Passed it on to the future generations, make legislation to protect it."

Here "it" means specifically to the use of "fine needles to open up its *Jingmai*, regulate its *Qi* and blood, manage its junction of flow and counter flow and entering/exiting points."

The conviction among ancient Chinese medical experts that *Jingmai* treatment can and should be passed on generationally ranks as an important prophesy in the history of medicine, demonstrating the wisdom and courage of the early doctors who championed it. All the more unfortunate then that so many flawed interpretations (such as the one above) have been made in the name of this great text – interpretations that deprive future generations of their promised legacy, and that promote the compromised system of acupuncture that is practiced so widely today.

4、三"其"

"其"字是个代词，特指他、他们、他们的；那、那个、那些……写该段经文，为了简明扼要，一连用了三个"其"字，代表病证（含病证的部位）。

如"欲以微针通其经脉"，即是指用微针（含毫针）刺支配病证和与病证相关的经脉。"调其血气"，即指调整病证（含病证的部位）的血气。"营其逆顺出入之会"，即指营支配病证和与病证相关的经脉。

据此破解可知，该段经文描述的针刺经脉，绝对不是在全身盲目乱刺，而是先明确诊断，确定病证的部位，特在支配该病证和与该病证相关的经脉上针刺，调整症证（含病证部位）的血气，增加支配病证和与病证相关经脉的功能，达到治病目的。遗憾的是，在过去的破解中，常常忘记这些代表主语的"其"字，由此使经文走了样，变了味，致使后人理解难，承用更难。

5、"令可传于后世，必明为之法。"

"令可传于后世，必明为之法。"

专指"微针通其经脉，调其血气，营其逆顺出入之会"而言，与其它无关。

它明确指出，该法及理论一定能传于后世，应写书、立法传承。这个描述既倾吐了中国古代医学家，对针刺经脉治病的伟大预言，又显示了他们驰骋纵横，视死如归的精神。但遗憾的是，多少年来一直没有把该段经文破解正确，当然也就无法将其如实传于后代了。也由此使中国的针刺经脉治病才形成目前的状况，最少是重要原因之一。

Furthermore, we know that the sentences "Use fine needles to open up its *Jingmai*, regulate its *Qi* and blood, manage its junction of flow and counter flow and entering/exiting points" and "Passed it on to the future generations, make legislation to protect it" are highly specialized interpretations written in a kind of technical language of the time. If readers are not equipped with clinical knowledge of this language and not experienced in related research, they will never penetrate the meaning of the text in an accurate way. Indeed, in order to interpret these writings accurately it is necessary to understand the meaning of this technical language along with every detail of its special symbolism. Additionally, the text is written in a question and answer form, and each part is correlated (to every other part), making it a unified whole. For this reason, if interested parties are to interpret this writing correctly they need to read the entire text thoroughly and study the inter-relationships between each part – this, rather than simply reading random or isolated paragraphs.

(C) The special value and significance

This text has extraordinary value and great significance, for it accurately summarizes the method of using different types of needles to acupuncture different tissues in the body. This passage affirms the medical wisdom of using fine needles to pierce the most sensitive parts of the body i.e., the *Jingmai*. In clinical practice it advocates the use of subtle instruments such as (in today's world) fine filiform needles that gently pierce the *Jingmai* and generate immediate responses (the arrival of *Qi*), thus achieving effective healing. The text also explains the healing mechanism of acupuncture *Jingmai* for managing *Qi* and blood of the body parts that contain disease. The term "*shun ni chu ru zhi hui*" further explains the workings of the *Jingmai* and confirms the fact that using fine needles in acupuncture can make the *Jingmai* stronger. (Interestingly, the text compares the process of transformation of a patient receiving acupuncture to the emergence of a butterfly from a cacoon.) In the process it helps acupuncture make the leap into the modern world of scientific theory – just as it was foretold long ago.

由此而知，"欲以微针通其经脉，调其血气，营其逆顺出入之会。令可传于后世，必明为之法。"专业性很强，用的全是针刺经脉治病的专业术语，和代表科研成果的特殊词汇。因此，如果没有针刺经脉治病的临床实践经验，和扎实的相关科研功底，就永远不会破解。只有懂得这些含意，了解每个细节，才能正确破解。再加上该篇经文，是问答式的特殊结构，整篇文章相互连贯，丝丝如扣，浑然一体。为此要想破解该段经文，仅读该段经文是不够的，只有通读，熟读整篇文章后，并进行深入研究，认真分析相互间的关系，才能真正破解其意。

（三）特殊价值和意义

该段经文价值非凡，意义重大。因为其认真总结了前 2500 年，用多种针在躯肢不同组织，针刺治病的方法和经验。特别肯定了用微针在躯肢最敏感的组织——经脉上，针刺治疗病证的奇法。这种方法，即是用毫针等微针，轻轻刺在躯肢的经脉上（中），就立刻能引起明显的反应（气至），并可获得较好的疗效。确立了针刺经脉治病，是通过被刺的经脉，调整病证（含病证的部位）血气治病的机理。利用了"逆顺出入之会"，表达躯肢经脉的方法。确认通过针刺经脉治病，能使被刺的经脉功能增强……使中国的针刺治病，经历了如同蛹化成蝶的特殊阶段，一举跨入方法绝妙，理论科学，疗效独特，理念先进的新时代。并预言此法及理论能世代相传，特撰写《灵枢》促使其实现。

From its origins *Ling Shu* was highly respected by doctors and generations of medical experts who developed it according to their own local perspectives. However, due to incorrect understanding and lack of seriousness acupuncture *Jingmai* was distorted in many ways. This is a great tragedy for Chinese acupuncture and has had catastrophic consequences on today's clinical practice (such as the use of fine needles to directly supplement *Qi* deficiency and drain *Qi* excess). Also in error is the theory that considers the *Jingmai* to be a unique system different and separate from the actual nerves and vessels of the nervous system. What creates such misapprehensions? Generally speaking, a partial and incomplete reading of the text. In order to address this problem and associated issues, we should use the given text to deal with related problems, a task that in the end should prove relatively easy. However, if we try to address the current situation and related problems with other methods, we will find these methods useless. This, in a nutshell, shows the relevance and great value of the ancient text we are dealing with.

In short, the text shines with the wisdom of the ancients and with their hope and firm belief in the healing power of the *Jingmai*. This work is a milestone, a fossil museum, and an exhibition hall rolled into one. Indeed, unless you read it attentively you will never truly understand Chinese acupuncture and the purpose/meaning of the *Ling Shu*. Motivated students should read this text often, strive to understand it correctly, and take it deeply to heart so that they can help restore its original teachings and make it better serve the goals of modern healing practice everywhere.

III. "A poor doctor only looks for the physical location of an acupoint, while a superior doctor seeks the spirit (*Shen*)." The spirit" mentioned here is wondrous; it is like a distinguished guest entering our door; without seeing the disease, how can one know the cause?"

Ling Shu - Nine Needles and Twelve Yuan-Source Points says: "A poor doctor only looks for the physical location of an acupoint, while a superior doctor seeks the spirit (*Shen*) in the point. The spirit is wondrous; it is like a distinguished guest entering our door; without seeing the disease, how can one know the cause?"

Although this text is taken from the *Nine Needles and Twelve Source Points* it was written earlier than the *Ling Shu*. See Chapter 3 for a detailed interpretation.

《灵枢》闻世后，医学专家们非常崇拜，历代医学家，从不同角度传承发展。但是，因为没有正确认识和认真对待该段经文，使针刺经脉治病，在某些方面已偏离轨迹，沿着变异方向发展。这是中国针刺经脉治病的一大悲剧，也由此引起了灾难性的后果。如当今在临床上常用的用针直接补虚证、泻实证的技术、经脉是有别于神经，血管，至今还未找到的独特系统……使被针刺治病数千年的经脉，变的悬疑叠起，陷入困境，就是部分佐证。要想纠正目前的状况，解决相关问题，只要运用该段经文，直击有关问题，将会易如反掌。相反，想采用其它方法解决相关问题，及目前处境，将会苍白无力，黯然失色。这也正是该段经文的现实意义和重要价值。

简而言之，该段经文精彩绝伦。它不仅闪烁着中国古代医学专家们的智慧，而且凝聚着他们献身于中国医学的伟大理想和坚定信念。它既是一个里程碑，又像是一个化石库、展览馆……如果没有读懂它，就不会真正明白中国的针刺经脉治病，更不会知道写《灵枢》的目的和意义。因此，我们一定要熟读该段经文，并正确认识、认真对待。使中国的针刺经脉治病，恢复本来面貌，发挥更大作用，更好地为人类健康服务。

三、读"……粗守形，上守神；神乎神，客在门；未睹其疾，恶知其原。"之感悟

《灵枢·九针十二原第一》曰："……粗守形，上守神；神乎神，客在门；未睹其疾，恶知其原。"该段经文。

虽出于《九针十二原第一》，但早于《灵枢·小针解第三》，因其对该段经文进行详细解读。

I think the interpretation of the *Ling Shu*, Chapter 3 is largely incorrect. It completely contradicts the meaning of the original passage.

"A poor doctor only looks for the physical location of an acupoint, while a superior doctor seeks the spirit (*Shen*)" means that a poor doctor only knows how to apply needles to the acupuncture points, while a superior doctor knows how to acupuncture the *Jingmai* within these points – the somatic nerves.

"The spirit is wondrous; it is like a distinguised guest in the door" means that *Shen* is very mysterious; it is like an honored guest who resides within the points themselves. The *Shen* mentioned in this passage actually refers to *Jingmai*-the somatic nerves. "Without seeing the disease, how can one know the cause?" means that if a doctor does not observe and understand a particular disease he can never understand the origins of that disease.

T.N. Chan Interpretation: Based on observations made by Dr. Jiao, it could be said that the ancient Chinese system of Jingmai is more or less equivalent to the modern concept of the human nervous system. As such, this system plays a central part in linking up the physical body to the Divine Matrix or Higher Intelligence – the Tao, if you will. Critical to this connection is the Shen mentioned above and throughout the following text. The Shen, which means "spirit" or "diety," is also one of the three fundamental life energies, along with Qi and Jing. Shen flows into us, out of us, through us, and around us, connecting us to the universe and representing, as it were, the divine plasma that we are all engulfed in, as well as the divine force that dwells within each living person. In other words, we are all made up of the same stardust materials that originated in an infinitesimally small space the size of a quark at the moment of the Big Bang.

It can be said that just as we could connect to the Internet through WiFi to anywhere in the world, we could connect to the Divine Matrix through our Shen. "Where is the Internet?" one might be asked. "Where is this digital information we can access at any time with a simple username and password?" Answer: It is nowhere, yet it is everywhere. It is all around us, like the Spirit or Shen itself. This means, in turn, that when acupuncturists insert a needle into one of the Jingmai points, this needle serves to "download" cosmic healing Shen into a patient's body, much in the way that digital messages are downloaded by WiFi onto our personal computers. This "download" is made possible since the Jingmai interfaces the physical with the etheric. In other words, the Divine Matrix is not only outside of us in the cosmos, but inside of us in the very network of neurons that weaves its way throughout our bodies; it is the acupuncture needle that connects the two. As the Chinese sages have always maintained, "All things in the universe are interrelated."

我认为《灵枢·小针解第三》对其破解是错误的，完全违背了经文的原意。

"粗守形，上守神"，即是低劣的医生只知道针刺穴位治病，而高明的医生则知道在穴位中针刺经脉（神经躯肢）治病。

"神乎神，客在门"，即是说"神"非常神奇，像贵客一样位于穴位之中。文中所称"神"实指"经脉"（躯肢神经）。"未睹其疾，恶知其原"。即是说，没有看懂疾病，怎么能知道病因。

Based on the content of this writing, it is estimated that it may have been written as long as 3,000 years ago. According to this notion, Chinese medical experts knew how to find the *Jingmai* within the acupuncture points – the somatic nerves – using fine needle acupuncture almost before the invention of written language.

IV. Analysis of "A poor doctor only knows how to look for the physical joints (*Guan*) while the superior doctor knows how to find the gate mechanism in the point (*Ji*)... This is the complete explanation of the *Tao* of acupuncture."

Ling Shu Chapter 1 - Nine Needles and Twelve Source Points says: "A poor doctor only knows how to look for the physical joints (*Guan*) while the superior doctor knows how to find the gate mechanism in the point (*Ji*). The movement of *Ji* never exceeds its space. When we observe it from the outside, *Ji* activity appears tranquil in the space it occupies. It appears to have only a slight movement. Its coming cannot be met and its going cannot be followed or grasped. Those who understand the gate mechanism are able to pierce the points precisely without missing a hair's breadth. Those who do not understand the gate mechanism will miss the timing of *Qi*. Piercing points in a random way is useless. Knowing where *Qi* is coming from and where it is going and timing of *Qi* to get the best result is important. This phenomenon is really wondrous. The poor doctor remains in the dark (about it), while the superior doctor knows all these (important facts). When *Qi* goes away, it is called 'counter flow'; when it arrives, it is called 'flow.' When counter flow and flow are grasped, positive actions can be practiced without question. If you meet (counter) *Qi* and deplete it, how can the excess not be drained? Follow and reinforce it, how can the deficiency not be filled? Countering and following the *Qi*, following the *Qi* dynamics with one's mind, this is the complete explanation of the *Tao* of acupuncture."

诠释内容推测，该段经文最低出现在 3000 年前。据此证明，中国医学专家，早在3000年前，就运用毫针在穴位中刺经脉（躯肢神经）治病了。

四、解析"粗守关，上守机……针道毕矣。"

《灵枢·九针十二原第一》曰："粗守关，上守机。机之动，不离其空。空中之机，清静而微。其来不可逢，其往不可追。知机之道者，不可挂以发。不知机道，叩之不发。知其往来，要与之期。粗之暗乎，妙哉！工独有之。往者为逆，来者为顺。明知逆顺，正行无问。迎（逆）而夺之，恶得无虚。追而济之，恶得无实。迎之随之，以意和之。针道毕矣。"

Although this scripture is from the *Ling Shu* its origin dates back to an earlier time. This fact is explained in detail in *Ling Shu Chapter 3 - Explanation of Small Needles*. Generations of doctors have tried to interpret this passage, but most never considered perspectives outside the framework of *Ling Shu Chapter 3 - Explanation of Small Needles*. When I checked the original scripture I found that the interpretation was patently incorrect. Indeed, some interpretations directly contradicted the original meaning of the passage. If the study of acupuncture follows these erroneous interpretations, the passage "A poor doctor only knows to look for the physical joints (*Guan*) while the superior doctor knows how to find the gate mechanism (*Ji*). This is the complete explanation of the *Tao* of acupuncture" would be burdened with mistakes and never be accurately revealed to the world. Therefore, only the interpretation based on the true meaning of the text can return the valuable information and scientific research embodied in this text to its rightful place in Chinese acupuncture theory.

The following are interpretations based on the original meaning of the text: "A poor doctor only knows to look for the physical joints (*Guan*) while the superior doctor knows how to find the gate mechanism in the point (*Ji*)" means that a poor doctor treats disease only by working with the physical acupuncture points, while a superior doctor knows how to treat diseases by acupuncturing the *Ji* within these points. "The movement of *Ji* never exceeds its space" means that *Ji* itself (inside the space) can move, but its movement never exceeds its space. This interpretation calls our attention to the fact that *Ji* is specified as an object (or tissue); it is definitely not *Qi*. The term "*Kong*" does not mean points because the movement of *Ji* does not exceed its space. "Its" refers to *Ji* itself. Thus "never exceeds its space" means that *Ji* does not leave its space (area). "When we observe it from the outside *Ji* activity appears tranquil in the space it occupies. It appears to have only a slight movement" means that *Ji* is in its space. It appears to be quiescent when observed from the outside, and its movement is very subtle (this conclusion is probably derived from anatomy and the direct examination of *Ji*).

该段经文虽出于《灵枢·九针十二原第一》，但是源于更早，因在《灵枢·小针解第三》即有详细解读。后世的破解，一直没有摆脱《小针解第三》的框架。后来，我在认真核对原文时发现《小针解第三》诠释经文有误，其中有些内容完全违背了原意。如果在针灸学中，刻意沿用其诠释，将会使"粗守关，上守机……针道毕矣。"沉陷在错误诠释之中，永无见天之日。所以，只有根据该段经文的真实含意进行诠释，才能使可贵经验和重大科研成果，重新屹立在中国针刺经脉治病中。

　　现据经文原意诠释如下："粗守关，上守机。"即是说低劣的医生只知死守穴位治病；而高明的医生则知道在穴位中刺"机"治病。"机之动，不离其空。"即是说"机"本身（内部）能活动，但活动范围不离开它的空间。这样破解说明"机"特指一种物体（或称组织），绝对不是气。"空"不是指穴位。因"机"之动，不离其空。"其"当然应指"机"本身。所以，不离其空，就是不离开它的空间（范围）。"空中之机，清静而微。"即是说"机"在其空间，从表面上看非常清静，仅有微微之动（这可能是通过解剖直接观察机的外形而得出的结论）。

"Its coming cannot be met and its going cannot be chased" means that in the space of *Ji* (inside the space) information can be transmitted in and out. This transmission is natural and wondrous – an observer could never observe its workings from the outside, a conclusion most likely derived from complicated physiological experiments. "Those who understand the gate mechanism are able to pierce the points precisely without missing a hair's breadth" means that those who understand the essence of *Ji* can pierce it without being off by a hair's breadth. "Those who do not understand the key point will miss the timing of *Ji*" means, metaphorically speaking, that those who do not understand the essence of *Ji* can – metaphorically speaking – pull the trigger but the gun will not shoot. In other words, if doctors do not understand the timing of *Ji*, and if they practice acupuncture only by randomly piercing the points they will never master their art. "Knowing where it is coming from, where it is going and the timing *Qi* to get the best results are all important" means that if doctors know the coming and going of *Qi* they will easily pierce *Ji*. "This phenomenon is really wondrous. The inferior doctor remains in the dark, while the superior doctor knows all these (important facts)" means that inferior doctors cannot understand the ways and means of acupuncture practice in a deep way; only superior doctors can plumb its subtle secrets.

"When *Qi* goes away, it is called counter flow; when it arrives, it is called flow. When counter flow and flow are grasped, positive (healing) actions can be taken without (doubts or) questions" means that the direction that is contrary to the "arrival of *Qi*" is the direction of counter flow, while the direction of the "arrival of *Qi*" is the direction of flow. Knowing the meaning of flow and counter flow, one can boldly practice acupuncture with no further questions. "(If you) meet (counter) *Qi* and deplete it, how can the excess not be drained? Follow and reinforce it, how can the deficiency not be filled?" means that if we counter the arrival of *Qi* and drain it, how can we avoid weakening the "arrival of *Qi*"? If we chase and push in, how can we not strengthen the "arrival of *Qi*"? "Countering and following the *Qi*, following the *Qi* dynamics with one's mind" means that by pushing in the needle and pulling it out we can adjust the intensity of the "arrival of *Qi*". "This is the complete explanation of the *Tao* of acupuncture" means that the above dictums are all basic to the correct practice of basic acupuncture.

"其来不可逢，其往不可追。"即是说在机之空间（内部），往返传递信息，自由而神奇，客观根本无法感知（这可能是通过复杂的生理试验而得出的结论）。"知机之道者，不可挂以发。"即是说，知道机的要意，就能毫发不差的刺中它。"不知机道，叩之不发。"即是说，不知道机的要害，就是叩了扳机，也等于没有发。也就是说，不懂机的要意，乱刺是刺不中的。"知其往来，要与之期。"即是说知道其来拢去脉，就易刺中"机"。"粗之暗乎，妙哉！工独有之。"即是说低劣的医生，什么也看不见，只有高明的医生，才能领悟到其中的奥妙。

　　"往者为逆，来者为顺；明知逆顺，正行无问。"即是说，在针刺时能使"气至"消退的方向为逆，能使"气至"来的方向为顺；知道逆顺之意，就大胆去刺，不要再问了。"迎（逆）而夺之，恶得无虚；追而济之，恶得无实。"即是说，运用迎使气夺的方法，还能不使"气至"减弱吗？运用推而进的方法，还能不使"气至"增加吗？"迎之随之，以意和之。"即是说，将针迎和随（退和进），就可随意调整"气至"的强度。"针道毕矣。"即是说针刺的道理就是这些了。

According to the interpretation of the above passage, we know that as early as 3,000 years ago Chinese medical experts used the word "*Ji*" in the proper context and had a deep understanding of its meaning. Also, that the superior doctors knows how to treat disease by piercing the *Ji* within the points. When it comes to piercing with needles, the direction that can trigger the "arrival of *Qi*" is the correct direction, while the direction that weakens the "arrival of *Qi*" is the wrong direction. Finally, the methods of "Meet" and "Chase" can be used to adjust the intensity of the "arrival of *Qi*."

Medical experts in ancient China described *Ji* in a vivid and mysterious way. But what is *Ji*, really? According to studies and to knowledge of modern anatomy and physiology, it is clear that the somatic nerves are in many ways astonishingly similar to the *Ji* described by ancient Chinese medical experts. Therefore, we can assume that as early as 3,000 years ago Chinese medical practitioners had systematically summarized their technique of using fine needles to stimulate the somatic nerves. Even today such skill and wisdom ranks high in the annals of world medicine. At a time, when the level of medical practice throughout the world was still primitive and people knew very little about the structure of the human body, ancient Chinese doctors were intimately familiar with the workings of the somatic nerves, and were busy inventing scientific techniques to treat a host of human diseases.

The above facts fill me with awe and make me deeply appreciate the wisdom, passion, devotion and nobility of ancient Chinese medical experts. In essence, what they explored was a miraculous path of heaven. As early as 3,000 years ago they used Chinese needling techniques to lead them into the heaven realm of science. For this reason, we must understand their heritage correctly, and pass it on to coming generations with great sincerity.

Truth is the most important thing.

Comments on whether the medical art of Chinese needling is scientific should be based on facts. The analysis of the passage "A poor doctor only knows to look for the physical joints (*Guan*) while the superior doctor knows how to find *Ji* – the gate mechanism. This is the complete explanation of the Tao of acupuncture" has proved from one perspective that Chinese needling practice is indeed scientific.

据诠释经文之意推知，中国医学专家，早在 3000 年前就巧妙运用"机"字，并深刻理解"机"字的内涵。高明的医生则知道在穴位中刺"机"治病。在针刺时，只要能使"气至"出现的方向即为正确方向，反之则为逆的方向。并运用迎和随的方法调整"气至"的强度。

中国古代医学家，将"机"描述的生动而神奇。那么，"机"究竟指什么？根据针刺试验、现代神经解剖、生理知识，对比分析发现躯肢的周围神经，与古代医学家描述的"机"，在多方面惊人相似。由此推知，中国医学专家，早在 3000 年前，就通过精湛神经解剖、生理知识和针刺躯肢治病的实践经验，系统总结出在全身穴位中，针刺躯肢神经治疗病证的特殊技术和经验。这些都是中国古代医学家们的伟大发现，和多学科的重大科研成果。他们在世界医学极端落后，对人体结构茫然无知，悬疑迭起的历史背景下，发现了人体的躯肢神经，并发明了运用毫针刺躯肢神经，治疗全身多种疾病的科学方法。

上述事实，使我感慨万千。进一步体会到中国古代医学专家们的聪慧、激情、执着、高尚。他们攀登的是一条神奇的天道。他们早在 3000 年前，就将中国的针刺治病，带进了科学的天堂。为此，我们必须正确认识，认真传承。

事实是最重要的。

评述中国的针刺治病是否科学，必须用事实说话。本文对"粗守关，上守机……针道毕矣。"的解析，即从一个侧面证明了中国针刺治病是非常科学的。

V. Analysis of "For those who practice acupuncture, (treat) deficiency by filling, excess by draining, chronic stagnation by eliminating and over abundance of evil *Qi* by withdrawing."

    Ling Shu Chapter 1 - Nine Needles and Twelve Source Points says: "For those who practice acupuncture, treat deficiency by filling, excess by draining, chronic stagnation by eliminating and over abundance of evil *Qi* by withdrawing." *Ling Shu Chapter 3 - Explanation of Small Needles* says: "Treat deficiency by filling." This phrase refers to using the fill method when there is deficiency at *Qi kou.* "(Treat) excess by draining" refers to using the draining method when there is excess at *Qi kou.* "Chronic stagnation by eliminating" means to eliminate the blood and tissues that have become corrupted. "Over abundance of evil *Qi* by withdrawing" tells us that if there is excessive activity in the *Jingmai* this means pathogenic factors are present. *Su Wen Chapter 54 - Explanation of Needles* says: "When the tip of the needle feels empty first and then solid this means there is heat under the needle, and that the solidness of *Qi* is caused by this heat" "M*an ze xie zhi*" means that when there is coldness under the needle a deficiency of *Qi* is present. "Chronic stagnation by eliminating" refers to letting out bad blood. "Abundance of evil *Qi* by withdrawing" means we do not press when pulling out the needle to let out the evil *Qi. Huang Di Nei Jing Ling Shu-Explained in Modern Chinese* [1] says: "The deficiency syndrome should be treated with the filling method so that the positive *Qi* can be supplemented. The full and excess syndrome should be treated with the draining method, so that the pathogenic factors of diseases can be eliminated. For symptoms caused by chronic stagnation of blood, the blood should be drained in order to eliminate the pathogenic factors that have stagnated in the body. For syndromes caused by the over-activity of pathogenic factors and pathogenic factors overcoming the positive factors, the draining method should be used to let out the pathogenic factors of disease, turning it from excess to emptiness."

---

[1] *Huang Di Nei Jing-Ling Shu Explained in Modern Chinese* Edited by Wang Hong Tu, People's Medical Publishing House 2006 First Edition.

五、析"凡用针者，虚则实之，满则泄之，宛陈则除之，邪胜则虚之。"

　　《灵枢·九针十二原第一》曰："凡用针者，虚则实之，满则泄之，宛陈则除之，邪胜则虚之。"《灵枢·小针解第三》曰："所谓虚则实之者，气口虚而当补之也。满则泄之者，气口盛而当泻之也。宛陈则除之者，去血脉也。邪胜则虚之者，言诸经有盛者，皆写其邪也。"《素问·针解篇第五十四》曰："刺虚则实之者，针下热也，气实乃热也。满而泄之者，针下寒也，气虚乃寒也。宛陈则除之者，出恶血也。邪盛则虚之者，出针勿按。"《黄帝内经灵枢·白话解》曰："属于虚证的，当用补法，使正气充实，属于满实证候的，当用泻法，以疏泄病邪；对于因血郁积日久而引起症状的，应当采用泻血法，以排除壅滞的病邪；对于病邪亢进，邪胜于正的，也应当采用泻法，以使邪气外泄，由实而虚。"（《黄帝内经·白话解》主编 王洪图 人民卫生出版社 2006 年第一版）

Different contemporary interpretations of *Huang Di Nei Jian-Ling Shu* tend to be similar because most are based on *Ling Shu - Explanation of Small Needles* Chapter 3. In fact, these interpretations are generally incorrect and totally distort the meaning of the original passage. In my opinion, the original meaning was derived by Chinese doctors, and from the experience and thoughtful reflection that comes from treating patients with fine needles (including filiform needles). When performing acupuncture, all doctors should insert the required needles at certain points on the body and then attempt to pierce the *Jingmai*. If the tip of the needle feels empty when it is pushed in (or soft, with little resistance, or again, with no special feeling), this is proof that the needle has not yet reached the *Jingmai*. At this time, one should pierce further in or change the direction and pierce again till the *Jingmai* is reached. When there is a sudden increase of resistance at the tip of the needle or a feeling of firmness, this sensation reflects the exact meaning of "(treat) deficiency by filling".

"(Treat) excess by draining" means when *De Qi* is too full it should be drained a little. *De Qi* is a phenomenon that ordinarily occurs when *Jingmai* is pierced. Sometimes if *De Qi* is too strong and the patient cannot bear the sensation, the doctor should withdraw the needle a bit so that *De Qi* is reduced. Based on the sentence "(Treat) excess by draining," the technique of adjusting the intensity of *De Qi* was conceived. "Chronic stagnation by eliminating" refers to the special sensation that occurs when the tip of the needle reaches (touches) the bones, tendons, or scar tissues and cannot penetrate any further. The appropriate action at this point is to withdraw the needle a little, change the direction, and then re-pierce the point. "Over abundance of evil *Qi* by withdrawing" refers to the severe shivering and numbness or pain that occurs when the needle pierces the *Jingmai*. Patients usually cannot bear this sensation, and many medical experts view it as a sign that pathogenic factors are present. When this sensation occurs the doctor should withdraw the needle a little. The pathogenic factors will then be relieved. This is the original meaning of the sentence "over abundance of evil *Qi* by withdrawing."

I think this interpretation not only matches the original meaning of the passage but clearly describes the core method of using fine needles to treat disease. Time flies like a weaver's shuttle and the world has experienced great changes. Even though 3,000 years have passed, these clinical techniques are still used on a regular basis by Chinese physicians. Thus, this passage not only has great scientific value but offers important medical advice that all modern practitioners would be wise to follow.

当代不同版本对其解读类同，均按《小针解第三》之意进行诠释。其实，这类破解都是错误的，完全违背了经文的本意。我认为经文的原意是临床实践家，用微（含毫针）针在躯肢特定部位（相对固定针刺点），针刺经脉治病的特殊技术和经验（感悟）。即凡在针刺时，每个人都应先将针在躯肢特定部位刺入皮下，然后再寻找针刺经脉。如将针往进推时，针尖处为空虚感（感松、阻力小、无特殊感觉），证明没有刺中经脉，此时应继续往进刺，或改变方向再刺，直到刺中经脉（针尖处阻力突然增大，有特殊感觉）为实。这即是"虚则实之"的确切含意。

"满则泄之"即指"得气"太满应泄出部分。因在针刺中经脉时必出现"得气"，有时因"得气"太强病人难以忍受，这时将针微往外拔一点，即可使"得气"减轻。由此即出现了"满则泄之"调整"得气"程度的技术。"宛陈则除之"是指在针刺时，针尖碰（触）到骨、肌腱、疤痕等时，再刺不进去的特殊感觉。解除之法，是将针稍往后退，改变方向再刺。"邪胜则虚之，"即指在针刺中经脉时，出现严重抽麻、疼痛等感觉，病人难以忍受，古代医学家视此现象为邪胜。这时应将针微往后退，邪胜即可缓解，这即是"邪胜则虚之"的本意。

我认为这样诠释，不仅符合经文原意，而且揭示了毫针刺经脉治病的核心技术。日月如梭，沧桑巨变，远隔三千年的今天，在针刺经脉治病的临床实践中，最常用的仍然是这类技术。所以，该段经文不仅有较高的科学价值，而且有重要的现实意义。必须大力弘扬，认真传承。

VI. New Understandings on "Slow then rapid is excess. Rapid then slow is deficiency."

Ling Shu Chapter 1 - Nine Needles and Twelve Source Points says: "'*The Great Essentials*' says: 'Slow then rapid is excess. Rapid then slow is deficiency.'" Based on this statement we know that this sentence is taken from *Ling Shu Chapter 1 - Nine Needles and Twelve Source Points*, and that its principles originated in a famous medical text called *The Great Essentials*. While there is no clear evidence of when *The Great Essentials* was written, many historical references, both ancient and modern, refer to it. Another important text *Su Wen* specifically mentions that *The Great Essentials* was, in fact, an ancient scripture. According to this reference, we can estimate that "Slow then rapid is excess. Rapid then slow is deficiency" embodies a very old concept and may well date from the ancient era.

Since the appearance of "Slow then rapid is excess. Rapid then slow is deficiency" in *The Great Essentials* medical experts have considered it to be of great importance. There are, however, different interpretations regarding its exact meaning, and it has influenced acupuncture technique in a number of different ways. Among them, *Ling Shu Chapter 3 - Explanation of Small Needles* says: "'Slow then rapid is excess' means insert the needle slowly and withdraw it rapidly. 'Rapid then slow is deficiency' means rapidly insert the needle and slowly withdraw it." This interpretation was then quoted relatively often, resulting in yet more deviations. It finally evolved into the "rapid and slow tonify and drain" method. This special method of "tonify the deficiency, drain the excess" was then passed down to the present day.

Among older medical texts there are different interpretations. For example, the text *Su Wen Chapter 54 - Explanation of Needles* says: "Slow then rapid is excess" which means withdraw the needle slowly and press it rapidly. Likewise, "Rapid then slow is deficiency" tells us to withdraw the needle rapidly and press it slowly.

六、读"徐而疾则实，疾而徐则虚"新悟

《灵枢·九针十二原第一》曰："《大要》曰：'徐而疾则实，疾而徐则虚。'"由此而知，该句经文出自《九针十二原第一》，源于《大要》。《大要》是什么年代形成，无据确证。多数书记载《大要》为古经篇名。《素问》有一处说：《大要》上古经法也。"据此推测"徐而疾则实，疾而徐则虚"非常古老，很有可能源于上古时期。

从《大要》"徐而疾则实，疾而徐则虚"闻世后，即引起医学专家们的高度重视。但对其确切含意，理解不同，由此对针刺技术产生过不同影响。其中《灵枢·小针解第三》曰："徐而疾则实者，言徐内而疾出也。疾而徐则虚者，言疾内而徐出也。"后世引用的比较多，变异比较大，最终演变成"徐疾补泻"法。这种特殊"补虚证，泻实证"的方法，一直流传至今。

在经文中，还有不同的破解，如《素问·针解篇第五十四》曰："徐而疾则实者，徐出针而疾按之。疾而徐则虚者，疾出针而徐按之。"即是佐证。

In my view, both of these interpretations are incorrect. Why? Because the sentences "Slow then rapid is excess. Rapid then slow is deficiency" do not actually describe how a doctor, while inserting and withdrawing needles, fills the deficiency and drains the excess through slow and rapid movement. Rather, it describes the particular experience of piercing points on certain parts of the body. Thus, according to the speed and intensity of resistance that suddenly occurs at the tip of the needle, one can tell if the *Jingmai* have been pierced or not. The mechanics of this method require the doctor to pierce the skin, then attempt to find and pierce the *Jingmai*. When the tip of the needle is about to reach the depth of *Jingmai*, the doctor gently pushs the needle in or gently twists it in. If a tightening feeling is felt at the tip of the needle, and if a sudden increase of resistance results, this means that the tip of the needle has successfully pierced the *Jingmai*, a sensation that is often referred to as "firm." When a doctor pushes the needle in or twists it in, and the feeling at the tip of the needle is soft or if there is little resistance despite the fact that the piercing speed is fast and hard, this means that the needle is still in the emptiness (that is, it has not yet pierced *Jingmai*), a condition that is referred to as "empty." Although thousands of years have passed, these sentences still offer the best advice for piercing the *Jingmai* and treating disease.

The Great Essentials describes the practice of piercing *Jingmai*. Through comparative studies of neuron-anatomy and knowledge of physiology and needling tests, it has been found that this practice is the same as that of piercing the somatic nerves.

According to this statement, we know that at a very ancient time Chinese medical experts began to use fine needles for treating disease, and that by so doing they accumulated valuable experience concerning whether or not to pierce the *Jingmai*.

我认为，上述两种诠释都是错误的。因"徐而疾则实，疾而徐则虚。"就根本不是描述依据进出针的徐疾，直接补虚证、泻实证。而是在躯肢特定部位针刺，根据针尖处出现（突然）阻力的速度和强度，判断是否刺中经脉的特殊经验。具体方法是，在特定部位先将针刺入皮下，然后寻找和针刺经脉。在针尖接近经脉的深度时，将针微往进推或捻转进针时，如针尖处突然变紧，即医生持针之手突然感阻力明显增加，就表示针尖已到实处（刺中经脉），简称实。如将针往进推或捻转进针，虽然速度快，用力大，针尖处仍感很松，即阻力较小，就表示针仍在虚处（未刺中经脉）简称虚。上述破解，才是经文的本意。几千年过去了，到目前为止，在针刺经脉治病中，该经验仍然为判断是否刺中经脉的最佳方法。

《大要》中描述的判断刺中经脉的经验，经与神经解剖、生理知识、结合针刺试验，对比分析后发现，该经验就是刺中躯肢神经的经验。

据此证明，中国医学专家，早在上古时期，即开始应用微针刺躯肢神经治病，而且积累了判断是否刺中躯肢神经的可贵经验。

VII. Analysis of "Pierce and *Qi* does not arrive, do not ask how many times; pierce and *Qi* arrives, remove the needle and no more piercing."

In *Ling Shu Chapter 1 - Nine Needles and Twelve Source Points* it says: "(If you) pierce and *Qi* does not arrive, do not ask how many times; pierce and *Qi* arrives, remove the needle and perform no more piercing" This means: (If you attempt to) pierce (the point) and *Qi* does not arrive, do not ask how many times (how many attempts you have made); (but if you) pierce the point and *Qi* arrives, remove the needle and perform no more piercings. The earliest interpretation on record of this scripture is in the *Huang Di Nei Jing Ling Shu - Notes and Elaborative Explanations* by Mr. Ma Shi, composed in the *Ming* Dynasty. He wrote: "If *Qi* does not arrive after piercing, one should not ask (how many) times but anticipate. It is like waiting for an honorable guest and not knowing that it is already sunset. If one pierces (the point) and *Qi* arrives immediately, remove the needle." The interpretations of future medical experts are mostly based on this passage.

I think this interpretation does not match the original meaning of the scripture. The phrase "Pierce and *Qi* does not arrive, do not ask how many times," specifically refers to "pierce." The text does not mention the terms "anticipate" or "wait." Mr. Ma Shi added the phrases "to anticipate" and also "it is like waiting for an honorable guest, one does not know it is already sunset." These latter additions are in my opinion superfluous and unnecessary. By including them the author not only failed to explain the text clearly but has violated its original meaning.

The fact is that between 2,500 and 3,000 years ago Chinese medical experts confirmed that if *Qi Zhi* (the "arrival of *Qi*") occurs when performing acupuncture with fine needles, healing effects will assuredly follow. Therefore, a number of efforts have been made to study this practice. Different techniques to trigger *Qi Zhi* have appeared over the years including those that focus on the number of times a piercing takes place (three times, six times, nine times, etc.), and those that focus on the depth that the needle reaches when piercing (shallow, medium, deep, etc.). Over the centuries, applying in-depth study and careful analysis, medical experts who were experienced in clinical practice finally concluded that "Pierce and *Qi* does not arrive, do not ask how many times; pierce and *Qi* arrives, remove the needle and do no more piercing" summarizes all the techniques that trigger *Qi Zhi*. Although this conclusion is based on experience, it is also clear that *Qi Zhi* is triggered by needling, not by waiting.

七、析"刺之而气不至，无问其数；刺之而气至，乃去之，勿复针。"

《灵枢·九针十二原第一》曰："刺之而气不至，无问其数；刺之而气至，乃去之，勿复针。"现查到《黄帝内经灵枢注证发微》（明·马莳著）"凡刺之而气尚未至，当无问其数以守之，所谓如待贵人，不知日暮者是也。若刺之而气已至，则乃去针耳。"后世医家多参考此文解读。

我认为这种破解不符合经文原意。因"刺之而气不至，无问其数"特论"刺"，并无"守"和"等"之意。马莳加"以守之"和"所谓如待贵人，不知日暮者是也"，完全是画蛇添足，多此一举。不仅没有解读清，反而违背了本意。

实情是，大约在2500-3000年间，中国医学专家已确认，用毫针刺穴位，如能出现"气至"，即可获得确信疗效。为此，大力研究针刺出现"气至"技术。由此即出现了不同的"气至"技术，如论针刺的次数（三、六、九等）深浅（浅、中、深）等候等多种出现"气至"的技术。大临床实践家、经深入研究，认真分析，最后才总结出可概括所有出现"气至"技术的方法，即是"刺之而气不至，无问其数；刺之而气至，乃去之，无复针。"这虽为经验之谈，但已明确了"气至"是用毫针刺出来的，而不是等候出来的。

When discussing the technique of using fine needles to treat disease, *Ling Shu Chapter 1 - Nine Needles and Twelve Yuan-Source Points* features this passage at the end. Today it is regarded as the sole standard that doctors should use when deciding whether or not to pierce *Jingmai*, and as such it represents the very core technique of needling *Jingmai*. Clinical practitioners cannot literally see the *Jingmai*, moreover; they can only estimate the location and depth of the nerves while piercing. If they miss the nerves on the first try, they should change the direction and depth, then pierce again till *Qi* arrives (which means that *Jingmai* is successfully pierced). Therefore, we can affirm the saying that "the arrival of *Qi* is the proof that *Jingmai* is pierced".

Due to different understandings of the text, different techniques have evolved over the centuries. After 2,500 years of this development the core technique of needling *Jingmai* (the phrase "Pierce and *Qi* does not arrive, do not ask how many times; pierce and *Qi* arrives, remove the needle and no more piercing.") has become one of many needling techniques. This evolution not only removed the technique from its core status, but made the *Jingmai* (somatic nerves) mysterious and incomprehensible.

Fortunately, clinical practitioners have always favored and preferred using this technique. Today it is not only in common use but is the best way to achieve assured healing effects in clinical practice.

If the status of this technique can be restored it will improve the healing effects in clinical practice and will benefit the discussion of needling *Jingmai* (somatic nerves) to treat disease.

VIII. Analysis of "The essence of needling is that once *Qi* arrives an effect is generated. This effect appears quickly, as when the wind is blowing away the clouds and the sky suddenly turns clear and blue. This process describes the complete *Tao* of needling."

Ling Shu Chapter 1 - Nine Needles and Twelve Source Points says: "The essence of needling is that once *Qi* arrives an effect is generated. This effect appears quickly, as if the wind is blowing away the clouds and the sky suddenly turns clear and blue. This process describes the complete *Tao* of needling."

《灵枢·九针十二原第一》在论述微针刺经脉治病技术时，特在最后选用该句经文。这一举措非常有价值。因其将该句经文当成判断是否刺中经脉的唯一标准和核心技术。因人体的经脉（躯肢神经），位于体表深部，临床实践家用眼睛看不见，只能估计经脉所在位置和深度而刺。如果一次没有刺中，改变角度和深度再刺，直到出现"气至"，即证明刺中经脉。因此，可以说："经脉若刺中，气至为佐证。"

认识不同，各自演变。2500 年过去了，针刺经脉的核心技术，"刺之而气不至，无问其数；刺之而气至，乃去之，无复针。"变成了多种针刺技术中的一种。这种演变，不仅使该方法失去了核心地位，而且使可被针刺中的经脉（躯肢神经），变的扑朔迷离，难认难解。

值得庆幸的是，临床实践家，一直热爱和喜欢运用该法。直到今日，该方法不仅一枝独秀，而且还是临床能取得确信疗效的最佳方法。

如能恢复该法的地位，不仅能提高临床疗效，而且对探讨针刺经脉（躯肢神经）治病颇为有益。

八、析"刺之要，气至而有效，效之信，若风之吹云，明乎若见苍天，刺之道毕矣。"

《灵枢·九针十二原第一》曰："刺之要，气至而有效；效之信，若风之吹云，明乎若见苍天，刺之道毕矣。"

"The essence of needling is that once *Qi* arrives an effect is generated" means that the most essential point to note about needling is that once the "arrival of *Qi*" occurs healing effects are assured. "This effect appears so quickly as when the wind blows away the clouds, the sky suddenly turns clear and blue" means that this healing effect is totally predictable, coming as quickly (and surely) as when the wind blows away the clouds and the sky suddenly becomes clear and blue. "This process describes the complete *Tao* of needling" means this is the basic principle of needling to treat disease, and that nothing else need be says (on the subject).

The text was originally written as a summary of needling practice. It describes in an affirmative way the best needling techniques for bringing about unique healing effects. The implied meaning is that this technique brings speedy and good healing, and that other methods pale in comparison.

Various understandings of the text evolved into different techniques of needling. After more than 2,000 years of this evolution the technique of needling *Jingmai* to trigger the "arrival of *Qi*" and achieve unique healing effects is still only one of many different needling procedures. This loss of the true understanding of *Jingmai* has reduced the healing effect of acupuncture, and has contributed to a severe deterioration in its clinical practice.

IX. Tentative Analysis of "Crossings of *Jie*, 365 junctions. For those who know the essence, one sentence is enough, while those who do *not* know talk pointlessly and endlessly. The so-called *Jie* are places where *Shen Qi* travels in and out; they are neither skin, muscles, tendons nor bones."

"刺之要，气至而有效，"即是说，针刺的要害，就是一旦出现"气至"就能获得疗效。"效之信，若风之吹云，明乎若见苍天，"即是说确信的疗效，如同风吹乌云散，立刻见晴天。"刺之道毕矣。"即是说针刺治病的道理就是这些，再没有说的了。

　　该段经文原为经验总结，用正说的方式描述了能获得独特疗效的最佳针刺技术。言外之意，即是说这种快而好疗效，其它方法皆黯然失色。

　　认识不同，理念演变。在两千多年后的今天，将刺中经脉出现"气至"，获得独特疗效的技术，变成多种针刺技术中的一种。由此，不仅严重影响了临床疗效，而且对躯肢经脉的认识也乱了方寸。

九、浅析 "节之交，365 会。知其要者，一言而终；不知其要，流散无穷。所言节者，神气之所游行出入也，非皮、肉、筋、骨也。"

Ling Shu Chapter1 - Nine Needles and Twelve Yuan-Source Points says: "Crossings of *Jie*, 365 junctions. For those who know the essence, one sentence is enough, while those who do *not* know talk pointlessly and endlessly. The so-called *Jie* are places where *Shen Qi* travels in and out; they are neither skin, muscles, tendons nor bones."[2] After this text was published medical practitioners used and interpreted it in many varying ways. Different interpretations of *Huang Di Nei Jing* mostly interpreted the *Jie* as "the gap in the articular cavity" or in "the physical joints." In my view, both these notions are incorrect. First, the text insists that, "they are not skin, muscles, tendons and bones." It also clearly points out that the *Jie* are not bones but something different. The physical joints and the articular cavities belong to the bone category, not to the skin, and because of this misunderstanding many interpretations are misleading and unconvincing. Second, it is incorrect to say that all of the 365 acupuncture points on the body are located in the gap of the articlular cavities. Many of these points (for example, *Cheng Shan, Cheng Jing, Zu San Li, Nei Guan, and Wai Guan*) are not in the gap of the articular cavities at all. Third, it is important to understand that the gap of the articular cavities is actually the place where *Shen Qi* (spirit energy) travels in and out. Moreover, there is mainly joint fluid in the joints, and it is an obvious impossibility that these fluids form junctions that allow the *Shen Qi* to travel in and out.

In order to interpret this text, we need to understand the basic meaning of *Jie* as well as its specific definition.

---

[2] 《黄帝内经灵枢诠释》南京中医学院中医系编著 上海科技出版社 1997 年 7 月第 5 次印。
Explanations of Huang Di Nei Jing-Ling Shu, edited and written by Department of Chinese Medicine, Nanjing University of Traditional Chinese Medicine, Shanghai Science and Technology Publishing House, July, 1997, fifth edition.

《灵枢•九针十二原第一》曰："节之交，365 会。知其要者，一言而终；不知其要，流散无穷。所言节者，神气之所游行出入也，非皮、肉、筋、骨也。"

　　（1）该段经文闻世后，很多医学家诠释承用。经查阅不同版本的《黄帝内经》，多将"节"破解成"关节腔间隙"或"关节"，我认为这类破解都是错误的。首先说，"非皮、肉、筋、骨也"之论述，明确肯定了"节"是骨以外之物，而关节、关节腔间隙仍属骨范畴。除此之外，还不能自圆其说。其一，365 个腧穴，均分布在关节腔间隙是不准确的。因很多腧穴（承山、承筋、足三里、内关、外关等），就根本不在关节腔间隙其二，关节腔间隙，为神气游行出入之处，令人难解。因关节腔中，主要为关节液，这些液体进行交叉形成会，再使神气游行出入，显然是不可能的。

　　要想正确破解该段经文，除弄懂"节"的基本含意外，还要注意经文对"节"的特殊界定。

This text can be divided into three parts. The first part tells us that "crossings of *Jie*, 365 junctions" (there are 365 crossings of *Jie*, or junctions). It is very difficult to understand that this is the core of the argument. The following two parts serve only to illustrate this first. The second part tells us that "For those who know the essence, one sentence is enough; those who do not know talk pointlessly and endlessly." This statement means that "crossings of *Jie*, 365 junctions" are extremely difficult to understand. Those who understand its essence will be able to explain it in one sentence. Those who do not will talk endlessly (but never reach the truth in the matter). The third part tells us that "The so-called *Jie* are places where *Shen Qi* travels in and out; they are neither skin, muscles, tendons nor bones." Translated, this sentence clearly explains that *Jie* are not muscles, skin, tendons and bones, and that they allow *Shen Qi* to travel in and out. What variety of tissue in the human body comprises this special tissue of *Jie*? Where is it located No one is certain. In order to find the *Jie* as described in the text, we must turn to anatomy and physiology, and make comparative studies of the tissues that are similar to *Jie* in terms of structure and function.

If such tissues can be found, we will then have proof that this text is entirely accurate, and thus we can verify its scientific value. I myself have found (in my own practice) that the anterolateral and posterolateral spinal tracts and neurofilments are, in fact, the *Jie* described in the text. Moreover, I have observed that the front and rear nerve roots (threads) join in sections, forming the front and rear roots. These two structures join and give shape of the spinal nerves which are similar to "Crossings of *Jie*" described in the text. Some of the spinal nerves pass through the foramen intervertebrales and then join together to form nerve plexus. They also converge and form different nerves that extend to the parts of the body that control various organs and tissues. Most of the nerves in the human body are capable of transmiting essential information (motion and sensory impulses) in and out, even though, as the text proclaims, they are not part of the skin, muscle, tendon and bone structures.

Long ago the famous Western physician Galen (130-200 AD) dissected a sheep and observed the structure of its brain. By so doing he discovered that there are empty "rooms" in the brain and "rooms" filled with fluids. This observation caused him to conclude that all sensations are recorded by the brain, and that all motions are triggered by this essential organ. Both, he believed, are caused by "fluids" flowing in and out of the brain. Galen's theory lasted for almost 1,500 years.

该段经文实为三段。第一段为"节之交，365 会。"也是核心段，因后两段都是说明第一段。第二段为"知其要者，一言而终；不知其要，流散无穷。"意为"节之交，365 会"非常难懂。如知道它的要害，一句话就说明白了；要是不知道其要害，就会漫无边际的乱说。第三段为"所言节者，神气之所游行出入也，非皮、肉、筋、骨也。"即是用一句话说清了"节"能使神气游行出入，又不是皮、肉、筋、骨。这样就将经文中描述的"节"，限定在既能交叉形成 365 会，又能使神气自由出入，还别于皮、肉、筋、骨的组织。"节"这个特定组织，究竟是人体的什么组织？具体在什么部位？全然不知。要想找到经文中描述的"节"，现在只能根据人体的解剖、生理知识等，对比分析在结构和功能，与"节"相似的组织。

　　如果能找到此类组织，不仅可以证明该段经文的真实性，而且可以进一步验证其科学价值。我发现，位于侧脊髓前外沟的神经根（细）丝和后外侧沟的神经根（细）丝，就是该段经文中描述的"节"。前、后神经根（细）丝，分别按节段进行交会，形成前根和后根，两根再相交形成脊神经的特殊形状，就与经文中描述的"节之交"非常相似。有些脊神经在出（入）椎间孔后，又会聚成神经丛。然后又经交叉、聚合等，形成不同的神经，分布在躯肢不同的部位，分别支配不同的器官和组织。分布在全身的各条神经，绝大多数都能自由传递出（入）信息（运动、感觉等），又不是皮、肉、筋、骨。

　　著名的医学家盖伦（Galen）（公元 130-200）切开羊脑后，发现脑是空的，在这些空心的腔室中有液体。他认为感知被大脑所记录，运动被大脑所启动，都是由体液通过神经到达脑室和离开脑室的流动而实现的。他的这种观点一直延续了将近 1500 年。

In 1751 a book titled *The Experiment and Observation of Electricity* proposed the theory that the human nervous system operates much like a network of "electrical cables" carrying electrical impulses to and fro throughout the body. Fifty years after publication of this book the Italian scientist Luigi Calvani and the German biologist Emil du Bois-Regmend proved that when electric impulses are sent through various nerves they stimulate tremors in the muscles. It was also discovered that the brain itself is capable of generating electrical impulses. These findings replaced Galen's theory that nerves connect to the brain via the in-flow and out-flow of fluids.

T. N. Chan Interpretation: Although some argue that when Galen spoke of "fluids," he actually refered to what we know to be Qi or energy flow.

Around 1810, the Scotsman Charles Bell observed that when he cut the back nerve roots (rear roots) and the abdominal nerve roots (front roots) of an experimental animal its muscles were paralyzed *only* if the nerve roots (front roots) in the abdomen were cut. In France, Francois Magendie then proved that the back nerve roots (rear roots) send sensory information into the spinal cord. Based on these discoveries, Bell and Magendie reasoned that the human nervous system is indeed similar to a set of electrical cables, but that some of these cables send information into the spinal cord and brain, and some send information out to the muscles. They observed that the anterior spinal roots contain only motor fibers, and that the posterior roots have only sensory fibers. They also proved that for each sensory nerve and motion nerve, the transmission of information runs exclusively *one way*. Finally, they showed that for most of their length the two types of nerves are wrapped together, separating only when they enter or leave the spinal cord. [3]

T. N. Chan Interpretation: The above historical facts show clearly that as early as the 18th century Western doctors knew that the front and rear nerve roots of the spinal cord and surrounding nerves transmit motional and sensory information. Today most books and atlases in neuron-anatomy published in the 20th century include detailed descriptions of the anterolateral and posterolateral spinal tracts and neurofilments.

---

[3] 《神经科学——探索脑》[美]Mark F Bear 等著，王建军主译 高等教育出版社 2004 年 7 月第 1 次印。
NEUROSCIENCE: Exploring the Brain by Mark F.Bear, Barry W.Connors, and Michael A.Paradiso. Translated by Wang Jian Jun, Higher Education Press, July, 2004, fifth edition.

1751 年一本《电的试验和观察》闻世了，提出了神经"电缆"论。后来在世纪之交，意大利科学家 Luigi Calvani 和德国生物学家 Emil du Bois-Regmend 证明，神经受到电刺激时会引起肌肉颤动，同时脑本身也可以产生电流。这些发现最终取代了"神经通过液体的流动而与脑相联系"的观点。

　　大约在 1810 年左右，Bell 通过切断动物的背根（后根）和腹根（前根），观察发现，仅切断腹根（前根），才会引起肌肉的麻痹。随后，Magendie 证实，背根（后根）将感觉信息传入到脊髓。Bell 和 Magendie 由此推论："每根神经都是电缆的复合体，其中一些纤维将信息传入到脊髓和脑，而另一些则将信息传送到肌肉。但是对于每一根感觉和运动神经纤维而言，信息传递则表现出严格的单方向性。这两类神经纤维在它们全长的大 部分都是包裹在一起的，只是当它们要进入或离开脊髓时才独立开来。

The above information demonstrates that several centuries ago Western doctors understood the root system of the spinal cord, as well as the fact that the peripheral nervous system has pathways that transmit motor and sensory information. In recent times, of couse, a great deal more scientific knowledge has been gained concerning the tracings in the anterolateral sulcus of spinal cord nerve roots (small) and posterior lateral sulcus of the nerve root (small).

All well and good. But it should also be pointed out that as early as 1,800 years ago medical experts in China, using anatomical and neuro-physical studies along with clinical observation, had already proved the existence of the sulcus of the spinal cord nerve roots (small) and the posterior lateral sulcus of the nerve root (thin) filament. They named these parts "Festival," theorizing that information is passed through the nerve roots (thin) fiber of the body from organ to organ. Early Chinese medical experts also observed the workings of the anterolateral and posterolateral spinal tracts and neurofilments, calling what they saw *Jie*. By so doing they confirmed that the somatic nerves transmit nerve information freely in and out along the anterolateral and posterolateral spinal tracts and neurofilments.

The "crossing of *Jie*" refer to the anterolateral and posterolateral spinal tracts and to the neurofilments. These tracts join together to form the front roots and the rear roots, ultimately combining to form the spinal nerves. After moving through multiple joints they turn into nerves in different parts of the body. The 365 acupuncture points that can be pierced are relatively fixed points on the somatic nerves. Therefore, ancient Chinese medical experts called them "Crossings of *Jie, 365* hui."

To sum up, the statement that "*Jie* are places where *Shen Qi* travels in and out; they are neither skin, muscles, tendons nor bones" presents a conclusive summary of Chinese medical experts' researches in neuron anatomy and physiology. These achievements are extraordinary and continue to have great value (for Chinese medicine). We must attach great importance to them, pass them on seriously (to future generations), and study them deeply in order to confront human disease in a fully scientific way.

上述资料证明，外国医学专家，真正搞清脊髓前根和后根，及周围神经传递运动和感觉信息的通路，只是百年前的事情。而在 20 世纪出版的有关神经解剖和图谱等书，多详细描记了位于脊髓前外侧沟的神经根（细）丝和后外侧沟的神经根（细）丝。

而中国医学专家，早在 1800 年前，就论证了在很久以前，通过解剖和神经生理研究，发现脊髓前外侧沟的神经根（细）丝和后外侧沟的神经根（细）丝，特称其为"节"。并明确肯定，躯肢神经传递出（入）信息，是分别通过"前神经根（细）丝和后神经根（细）丝，自由传递的。

"节之交"是指位于脊髓前外侧沟和后外侧沟的神经根（细）丝，相交形成前根和后根，再相交形成脊神经，多次相交后，分别形成躯肢不同部位的神经。在躯肢被刺的 365 个点，即是刺躯肢神经的相对固定点。所以，中国古代医学家，特将相对固定的 365 个针刺部位，称为"节之交，365 会。"

综上所述可知，"节之交，365 会。""所言节者，神气之所游行出入也，非皮、肉、筋、骨也"之论述，是中国医学专家，对神经解剖、神经生理等科研成果的总结论，成就巨大，价值非凡。我们必须高度重视，认真继承，深入研究，促使中国针刺经脉治病沿着科学道路，快速发展。

X. Reflections on "Observe the eyes; one can know (much from) their dilation and recovery."

Ling Shu Chapter 1 - Nine Needles and Twelve Source Points says: "Observe the eyes; one can know much from their dilation and recovery. *Ling Shu Chapter 3 - Explanation of Small Needles* interpreted this statement as meaning "The superior doctor knows how to observe the condition of the five organs by looking at the eyes. By knowing their size, examining whether they are slow moving or quick, smooth or astringent, one can tell where diseases are located." *Huang Di Nei Jing-Ling Shu Notes and Elaborative Explanations* (by Mr. Ma Shi, *Ming* dynasty) interpreted this statement as saying: "The situations of the five organs are revealed in the eyes. Therefore, if a superior doctor wants to know the patient's health status he will examine the eyes and will then know the disbursement and recovery of the positive *Qi*." Future generations often interpreted his words as meaning "examining the gaze (or look) in the eyes of a patient." In my opinion, this interpretation does not accord with the original meaning of the text. In my opinion, "Observe the eyes, one can know much from their dilation and recovery" means that by examining the eyes one will know the disbursement and recovery of the eye pupils. In this context, *San* means loosened, dispersed from aggregation, while *Fu* means recovery, replication, and repetition. (*The New Dictionary*, Jiling University Press, 2001, latest edition).

Modern medicine informs us that the pupils of our eyes are approximately the same size, that they are round and about ±0.3 cm in diameter. They are very sensitive to light, meaning that they shrink and dilate when stimulated by light of different intensities. In clinical examinations around the world it has always been known that when the pupils are simulated by relatively strong light they shrink, and that when the light source is removed they quickly recover their original size. The universal knowledge of these facts indicates that this method of diagnosing disease is not a modern invention, nor was it first used in the Western countries. Indeed, it was routinely used by ancient Chinese medical experts as long as 3,000 years ago. Unfortunately, due to incorrect interpretations through the centuries, it ended up buried and neglected in the text of the *Ling Shu - Nine Needles and Twelve Yuan-Source Points*, Chapter 1.

十、读"察其目，知其散复"之悟

《灵枢·九针十二原第一》曰："察其目，知其散复。"《灵枢·小针解第三》将其破解为"言上工知相五色于目，有知调尺寸大小缓急滑涩，以言所病也。"《黄帝内经灵枢注证发微》（明）马莳著、将其解读为"人之五色，皆现于目，故上工睹其色，必察其目，知其正气之散复。"后世多将其诠释为"观察病人眼神。"我认为上述破解均不符合经文原意。因"察其目，知其散复"是指检查眼睛知道瞳孔的扩散和恢复。因"散"有松开、分散、由聚集而分散……"复"有恢复、重复、反复等意（《新编字典》吉林大学出版社 2001 年最新版。）

现代医学可知，正常人的瞳孔等大、圆形，各 0.3CM±，对光反应灵敏。所谓对光反应，即是瞳孔受到不同强度光线的刺激，可出现收缩和扩散反应。在临床上检查光反应时，瞳孔因受较强光线的刺激，立刻引起收缩。待光源离开后，瞳孔即刻从扩散状，恢复到原来的状态。据此证明，依据瞳孔的对光反应，判断疾病的方法，不是现代人发明的，更不是西方国家先利用的。而是，中国古代医学专家，大约在 3000 年前就应用的常规诊断技术。遗憾的是，由于后世医学专家，对其破解有误，使其一直尘封于《灵枢·九针十二原第一》中。

In modern medicine, the shape and size of the eye pupils and their response to light are used for diagnosing disease and injury. For example, if both pupils are dilated and their response to light ceases entirely, a patient is presumed to be clinically dead. In case of brain injury cranial pressure increases due to the formation of intracranial hematoma, especially epidural hematoma. In this situation when the oculomotor nerves on the side of the injury are stimulated, the pupil on that side of the head shrinks. As the intracranial hematoma grows in size the oculomotor nerves are further pressed, leading to pupil dilation, decreased sensitivity to light, and in the worst case scenario total lack of response to light. If a clear diagnosis can be made during this period, and if the intracranial hematoma can be removed, the pressure to the oculomotor nerves is relieved and the size of the pupil and its response to light returns to normal.

If we can correctly understand and seriously utilize the statement "Observe the eyes, one can know much from their dilation and recovery," then we can significantly enhance the level of clinical diagnosis.

在现代医学中，将瞳孔的形状、大小和对光反应，当作判断死亡和诊断某些病损的重要依据。如双侧瞳孔散大，对光反应消失，即证明病人死亡。如在颅脑损伤时，因颅内血肿形成（特别是硬脑膜外血肿），颅压开始增高，当病变侧动眼神经受到刺激时，该侧瞳孔即开始缩小，随着血肿的增大，动眼神经受压，此时该侧的瞳孔即开始散大，对光反应减弱，直到消失。如能在此期间，明确诊断，彻底清除血肿，解除动眼神经的压迫，瞳孔的大小和对光反应即可恢复正常。

如果我们能正确认识和认真使用"察其目，知其散复"，将会大大提高诊病水平。

Chapter 2 - On *Jingmai*

Medical experts in China began to study *Jingmai* in the human body as early as 4,000 years ago. Over the years they made great advancements in scientific research through extensive, deep and persistent research.

Ling Shu Chapter 1 - Nine Needles and Twelve Source Points has made great contributions to the study of *Jingmai*. It not only correctly expresses and illustrates human *Jingmai*, it passes down an understanding of them from experience based on reflections, research, and scientific discussion. The following is a discussion on some of the important content in this passage.

Section 2.1 - *Jingmai* in the Spinal Cord

By means of an in-depth study of spinal cord *Jingmai* ancient Chinese medical scholars confirmed that they are an important part of the entire *Jingmai* system. The author of the *Ling Shu* believed that the *Jie* discussed in the text is actually the junction of somatic *Jingmai* and spinal *Jingmai*, similar in structure to the entrance and exit of somatic *Jingmai* at the spinal *Jingmai*. *(Ji Li* means inside the spinal cord.) Chinese medical experts discovered long ago that an important part of *Jingmai* is located inside the spinal cord. They called this area "spinal *Jingmai*" for short.

I. The Spine

As we know, the bones in the spine are among the most important structural elements in the human body. As early as two thousand years ago, they were identified and catalogued by Chinese medical experts, and over the centuries they have been studied extensively in many parts of China. For example, the *Ling Shu Chapter 14 - Gu Du (On the Measurement of Bones)*, informs us that: "There are two and half *Cun* between the hair line on the back of neck and the back bone; between the first thoracic vertebra process and the coccygeal vertebrae there are 21 spinal bones three *Chi* long. The upper part is 1.41 *Cun*[4], *Qi fen* is below, and thus the first seven spinal bones up to the first thoracic vertebra process are 9.87 *Cun* in length. This is the measurement of normal human bones. It is used to measure the length of *Jingmai*."

"DU LI – Inside Spinal Cord"
Calligraphy by Dr. Jiao

---

[4] one *Cun* is about 1.5 cm.

第二章 - 论经脉

中国医学专家们，早在 4000 年前即开始研究人体经脉了。后来，通过广泛、深入、持久研究，取得了巨大科研成果。

《灵枢·九针十二原第一》对经脉研究有重大贡献。它不仅用正确的方式表述和论证了人体经脉，使人体经脉从经验感悟跨入科学论断，而且开创了"微针刺经脉治病"的新时代。现摘重要内容进行论述。

第一节 - 脊里经脉

《灵枢·九针十二原第一》的作者，认真考究、深入研究，中国古代医学专家，对脊里经脉研究的成果。确认脊里经脉为人体经脉系统的重要组成部分。认为经文中表述的"节"，是躯肢经脉与脊里经脉的连接处，如同躯肢经脉在脊里经脉的出入口。脊里者，脊骨之里也。中国医学专家，早在很久以前，即发现了经脉的重要部分，就位于脊骨空里。所以，特称其为"脊里经脉"。

一、脊骨

脊骨是人体重要骨骼。早在两千多年前，中国医学专家就发现了，并进行了广泛而深入研究。《灵枢·骨度第十四》曰："项发以下至背骨长二寸半，膂骨以下至尾骶二十一节长三尺，上节长一寸四分分之一，奇分在下，故上七节至于膂骨九寸八分分之七，此众人骨之度也。所以立经脉之长短也。"即是佐证。

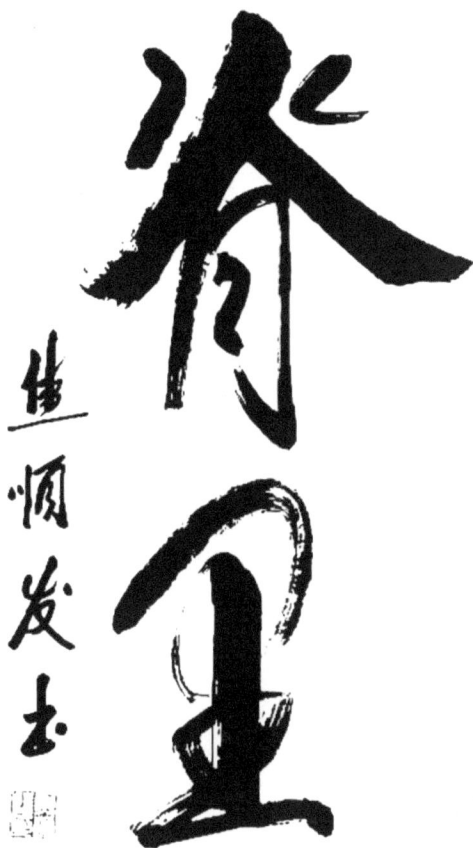

©ZL 200930124815.0

II. Hollow in the spine

Ancient Chinese medical experts have long known and studied the hollows in the middle of the spine, referring to them at times as "rooms." For example, the *Su Wen-Gu Kong Lun* (*On the Hollows of Bones*), Chapter 60, tells us that: "The top space of the spine is above *Feng Fu,* the bottom space of the spine is at the coccygeal vertebrae. The space inside the spine is between the two hollows."

III. *Jingmai* in the hollow inside the spine

Medical experts in China conducted in-depth research while studying the hollows inside the spine thousands of years ago, and in the process achieved profound and fruitful results. The results of this research are summarized below:

(A) The "Sui" of Jingmais

Ancient Chinese medical experts called the marrow in the hollow of the spine "*Sui.*" The text *Su Wen-Gu Kong Lun*, Chapter 60 says: "The hollow of *Sui* is located three *Fen* behind the brain, below the sharp bone at the rim of the skull. One of them is at the upper space of the spine above *Feng Fu.*" This passage likewise tells us that "The upper hollow of the spine above *Feng Fu*" is the space of *Sui.*" Also, that within this hollow is *Sui.*" The text *Ling Shu-Hai Lun* (*On the Sea*), Chapter 33 informs us that "There is a sea of *Sui* in the human" and "The brain is the sea of *Sui.*" This passage that informs us that *Sui* in the spaces of the spine is connected to the brain, which in turn is the sea of "*Sui.*"

二、脊骨空

中国古代医学家，早就发现了脊骨空。脊骨空即是脊骨中间的空。《素问·骨空论篇第六十》曰："脊骨上空在风府上，脊骨下空在尻骨下空。"即是佐证。知道脊骨上空和下空的位置，两空之间即是脊骨空。

三、脊骨空里经脉

中国医学专家早在数千年前，就对脊骨空里进行了广泛而深入研究，并取得了丰硕成果。现摘述于后：

（一）经脉之髓

中国古代医学专家称位于脊骨空里之物为"髓"。《素问·骨空论篇第六十》曰："髓空在脑后三分，在颅际锐骨之下……一在脊骨上空风府上。"这段经文描述的"脊骨上空风府上"为髓空，证明此空中即为"髓"。《灵枢·海论第三十三》曰："……人有髓海"、"脑为髓海……"证明位于脊骨空里的髓，上通脑为髓之海。

(B) The "Sea" of Jingmai

Chinese medical experts long ago described the hollows in the spine as being like the "sea" of *Jingmai*. Examples of this metaphor are found in the text *Ling Shu-Five Sounds and Five Tastes*, Chapter 65, which says: "*Chong mai* and *Ren mai* both start from the embryo; they go upward inside the back (backbone), which is the sea of *Jing Luo (Jingmai)*." The text *Zhen Jiu Jia Yi Jing - Qi Jing Ba Mai* or *A-B Classic of Acupuncture and Moxibustion*, Chapter 2 tells us that: "*Chong mai* and *Ren mai* both start from the embryo, then go upward inside the back (inside the backbone) which is the sea of *Jing Luo (Jingmai)*." When we read these passages we should pay special attention to the word "sea," which is described as the junction point where all the "rivers and streams" of the body converge. Only when we deeply comprehend the meaning of this symbol can we understand what is meant when the ancients said that *Jingmai* all over the human body converge into a central "sea."

(C) The Governor of Jingmai

Medical experts in ancient China discovered (and identified) the governor of *Jingmai* centuries ago. The word "*Du*" is a verb meaning to supervise, govern, monitor. Therefore, *Du mai* is the governor that supervises the other *Jingmai*. Many discussions about *Du mai* were collected in the text *Su Wen-Gu Kong Lun*, Chapter 60. *Nan Jing* conducted in-depth anatomical research on *Du mai* and found that it was located in the hollows inside the spinal column. The text *Nan Jing-Twenty-Eighth Nan* tells us: "*Du mai* starts from *Shu* point at the bottom of the spine, merges into the spinal column, goes upward to *Feng Fu*, and enters into the brain." (See Figure 2-4). In *Zhen Jiu Jia Yi Jing - Qi Jing Ba Mai,* Chapter 2 we read: "*Du mai* starts from the *Shu* point at the bottom of the spine, merges into the spinal column, goes upward to *Feng Fu*, and enters into the brain, its upper end goes to the nasal column, it is the sea of *Yang mai*." This passage not only borrowed the idea from *Nan Jing-Twenty-Eighth Nan* that *Du mai* is located in the space inside the spinal column; it also considered *Du m*ai to be the sea of *Yang mai*.

（二）经脉之海

中国古代医学专家，在很久以前就发现脊骨空里为经脉之海。《灵枢·五音五味第六十五》曰："冲脉任脉，皆起于胞中，上循背（背骨）里，为经络（脉）之海……"《针灸甲乙经·奇经八脉第二》曰："冲脉任脉者，皆起于胞中，上循脊里（脊骨之里），为经络（脉）之海。"即是佐证。读该段经文时，应特别注意"海"字。海为最大汇合，海纳百川即是恰当的描述。只有深刻理解海的含意，才能理解全身经脉汇于海的本意。

（三）经脉之督

中国古代医学专家，在很久以前即发现了经脉之督。因"督"字是个动词，有监督、监管、察看之意。所以，督脉即应是经脉监管之督。早在《素问·骨空论篇第六十》，就收集了很多关于督脉的论述。到《难经》对督脉进行了深入（解剖）研究，发现督脉就位于脊骨空里。《难经·二十八难》曰："然，督脉者，起于下极之俞，并于脊里，上至风府，入属于脑"（见图 2-4），即是佐证。《针灸甲乙经·奇经八脉第二》曰："督脉者，起于下极之俞，并于脊里，上至风府，入属于脑，上巅循至鼻柱，阳脉之海也。"该段经文不仅继承了《难经·二十八难》督脉位于脊骨空里，而且还认为督脉是阳脉（体表之脉）之海。

The discovery of *Du mai* represents a major leap forward for the understanding of *Jingmai* in the human body. It not only presents *Jingmai* as a complete system; it also provides doctors with the power to determine life and death, to regulate (energy flow), and to balance (human energies). The discovery of *Du mai* also contributed to passages in *Ling Shu - Nine Needles and Twelve Yuan-Source Points* such as: "Using fine needles to open up its *Jingmai*, regulate its blood and *Qi*, and manage its junctions of flow and counter flow, and entering and exiting points." In short, the discovery of *Du mai* made great contributions to the art of fine needle acupuncture.

(D) The Pivot of Jingmai

Around 2,000 years ago Chinese medical scientists discovered that there are pivots of *Jingmais* throughout the human body. The *Xuan Shu* point in *Zhen Jiu Jia Yi Jing* is the name of a point. It is located at the lower border of the thirteenth vertebra (the first lumbar vertebra). Precisely speaking, *Xuan Shu* is located below the lower border of the thirteenth vertebra. This discovery helps us better understand the *Jingmai* located inside the hollow of the spinal column.

督脉的发现，是认识人体经脉的一大飞跃。因为其不仅使经脉成了完整的系统，而且使其有了决死生、调平衡的功能。有了督脉，才会在《灵枢·九针十二原第一》中出现"欲以微针通其经脉，调其血气，营其逆顺出入之会"的论述。 总之，督脉对中国微针刺经脉治病贡献巨大。

（四）经脉之枢

中国医学家，大约在两千年前，即发现人体的经脉有"枢纽"。《针灸甲乙经·卷三》中的"悬枢"，虽然只是一个穴位名称，但其具体位于第十三椎节下间。确切的说，"悬枢"即是经脉的枢纽被悬吊在第十三椎节下间。这一发现，对认识位于脊骨空里经脉有特殊意义。

Generally speaking, as early as 2000 years ago medical scientists in ancient China had great success conducting in-depth research on the *Jingmai* inside the spinal column. According to ancient medical practitioners *Sui, Hai, Du, Shu* are all inside the hollw of the spine, and each has a special meaning. For example, *Sui* (marrow) describes the change of substance of *Jingmai* after *Jingmai* from all over the body enter the hollows of the spinal column. *Hai* (sea) describes how the *Jingmai* all over the body converge like numerous rivers on the hollow of the spinal column. *Du* (governor) describes how *Jingmai* all over the body converge into the hollow of spinal column, and how it governs the *Jingmai* throughout the entire body. *Shu* (pivot) refers to the marrow located on the lower border of the thirteenth vertebra inside the spinal column, and how it acts as a pivot for *Jingmai* all over the body. The above descriptions are clear and accurate. Unfortunately, over the centuries mistakes of interpretation have been made, causing the *Jingmai* inside the spinal column to become misunderstood by researchers.

IV. *Jie* of *Jingmai* inside the spinal column

"*Jie*"of *Jingmai* inside the spinal column is a new term, and this is the first time I have referred to it. Medical experts in ancient China discovered the *Jie* of *Jingmai* inside the spinal column centuries ago, and the information concerning it is very ancient. For example, in the ancient text *Zhen Jiu Jia Yi Jing-Zhen Dao*," Chapter 4, it says: "Crossings of Jie, 365 junctions. For those who know the essence, one sentence is enough; those who do *not* know talk pointlessly and endlessly. The so-called *Jie* are places where *Shen Qi* travels in and out; they are neither skin, muscles, tendons nor bones.*" Ling Shu Chapter 1 - Nine Needles and Twelve Source Points* made a great contribution to Chinese medicine by using this passage to summarize the somatic *Jingmai* and to discuss the location and special functions of *Jie*. After I read it I could see that the *Jie* described in this text is not located inside the physical joints or articular cavities. Instead, they are on both sides of the *Du mai* in the space of the spinal column. These *Jie* allow *Shen Qi* (spirit energy) to travel in and out, and as stated previously, they are *not* composed of skin, muscles, tendons or bones. Based on this concept, the *Jie* described by ancient Chinese medical experts is located inside the space of the spinal column. I refer to it as "*Jie* of *Jingmai* inside the spinal column."

"JIE of Jingmai – Inside Spinal Cord"
Calligraphy by Dr. Jiao

概括起来讲，中国古代医学家，早在两千年前，对脊骨空里的经脉，就从多个角度进行了深入研究，并取得了巨大成就。如古代医学家描述的髓、海、督、枢……虽都位于脊骨空里，但又各有特殊含意。如"髓"是重点描述了全身经脉进入脊骨空里后，经脉质的特征变化。"海"的描述，记录了全身经脉似百川汇聚于脊骨空里特征。"督"除描述全身经脉汇聚于脊骨空里外，还有统督全身经脉之意。"枢"指脊骨空里第十三椎节下间，被悬吊的髓，为全身经脉之枢纽。以上相关内容描记清楚，表述准确。但遗憾的是，在继承中对其原意破解有误，使脊骨空里的经脉悬疑叠起，迷茫难测。

四、脊骨空里经脉之节

"脊骨空里经脉之节"是个新词，我也是第一次使用。但其所表述的内容是很古老的。因中国医学家，在很久很久以前，即发现了脊骨空里经脉之节。《针灸甲乙经·针道第四》曰："节之交，凡 365 会。知其要者，一言而终；不知其要者，流散无穷。所言节者，神气之所游行出入也，非皮、肉、筋、骨也。"即是佐证。《灵枢·九针十二原第一》特别选用该段经文，用其概述躯肢经脉，论述"节"的位置和特殊功能。此举有重大贡献。我读该段经文后，认为经文中描述的"节"绝对不是位于"关节"或"关节腔"之内。而是位于脊骨空里督脉两侧。因为这些"节"，不仅能使神气所游行出入，而且又不是皮、肉、筋、骨。据此认为，中国古代医学家所描述的"节"，就位于脊骨空里，本人特称其为"脊骨空里经脉之节"。

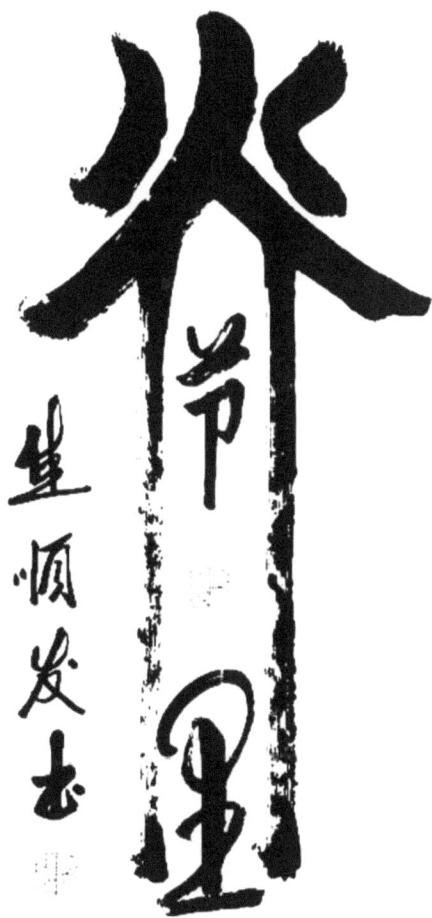

脊节里

生顺发书

©ZL 200930124815.0

There are many books that characterize *Jingmai* in such terms as *Jingmai, Jiu Juan, Zhen Jing* and similar words and phrases. Why then did *Ling Shu Chapter 1 - Nine Needles and Twelve Source Points* chose this particular passage? I think it was done deliberately. It is likely that the author of this work decided to use this passage after he verified the location and functions of *Jingmai* through anatomic and physiological experiments. Unfortunately, the generations that followed did not understand the original text, and they failed to correctly interpret the intent and objectives of its authors. They mistakenly located the *Jie* of *Jingmai* at the physical joints and articular cavities.Thus, the original meaning of *Jie* of *Jingmai* in the text of *Ling Shu Chapter 1 - Nine Needles and Twelve Source Points* fell into obscurity. This was, of course, a huge error. Because of it, the somatic *Jingmai* in the human body is not (understood to be) merged into the "sea," and the *Du mai* remains isolated and is not considered to be the "governor" of *Jingmai.* Up to this day these misinterpretations seriously hinder the application, research, and development of *Jingmai* theory.

Are the descriptions of ancient medical experts correct? Are my analysis and interpretations right? It is not helpful to make empty assertions. We can only rely on facts.

Our physical bodies today have the same structure and function they did in ancient times. Therefore, we need only compare the structure and function of our body's workings with descriptions that have come down to us from medical experts in the past to ascertain their accuracy.

Over the past 2,000 years medical science has developed in many significant ways. Today physicians are not only well versed in the anatomy and physiological functions of the human body; they are familiar with its micro-structures and complex functions, and can attain information on physiological matters simply by consulting modern medical texts. The materials inside the spinal column and the hollows in the column are located deep within the body; they can only be seen by direct anatomical observation. If we open a book on human anatomy we will find that the spinal column of the human skeleton supports the torso and the head (see Figure 2-1).

在《经脉》、《九卷》、《针经》……描述经脉的很多，表述的方式也不同。为什么《灵枢·九针十二原第一》只选该段经文呢？我认为这是其刻意这样做的。也可能《九针十二原第一》的作者，经过解剖、生理试验，进一步证实其位置和功能，才特意采用的。令人遗憾的是，后人没有读懂原文，更没有感受到《九针十二原第一》作者的意愿和目的，误将"经脉之节"定位于"关节"、"关节腔"……由此，使"经脉之节"的原意，一直尘封在《九针十二原第一》之中。这是一个重大失误。因该失误，一直使人体的躯肢经脉不能归入大海。督脉也一直孤独，始终无法统督全身之经脉，严重影响对经脉的应用、研究和发展。

古代医学家描述的是否正确？我分析和解读的是否对？绝不能凭空断言，只能靠事实说话。

现代人体的结构和功能，与古代人相同。所以，我们只要将现代人体相关的结构和功能，与古代医学家所描述的内容进行对比，即可证明其正确性。

在两千年后的今天，科学高度发达，医学家不仅知道，人体的大体解剖和生理功能，而且还知道微细结构和复杂功能。据此，我们只要翻开相关医学书，就可查到相关的内容和组织。脊骨和脊骨空里之物，均位于躯体的深部，只有通过解剖才能看见。翻开人体解剖学，在人体的骨架中，由脊柱支掌着躯干和头颅，详见图（2-1）。

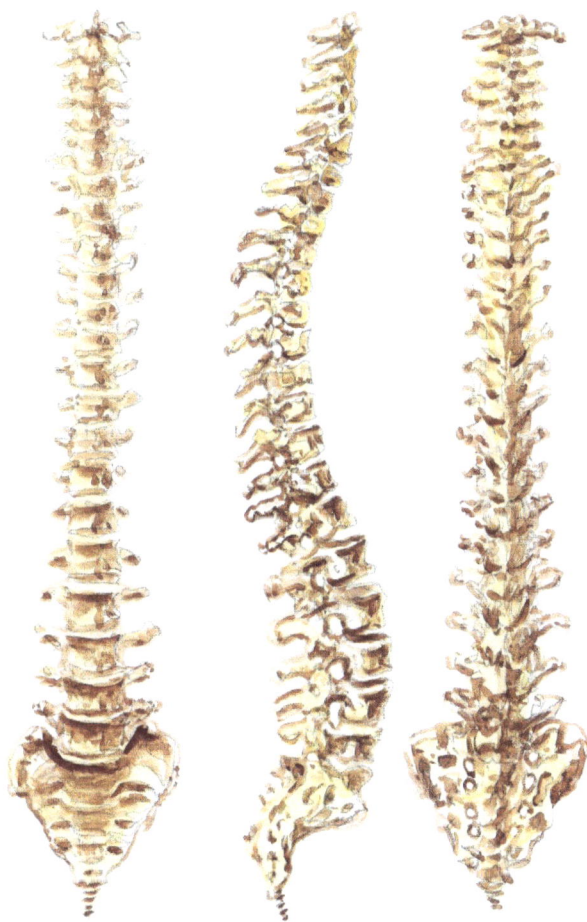

[2-1]

The human spinal column is described (in many texts) by ancient Chinese doctors (see Figure 2-2). Both the spinal column and the spinal ridge are part of the spine, and both have the same number of vertebrae. For example, there are seven cervical vertebrae on both, twelve thoracic vertebrae, five lumbar vertebrae, four sacral vertebrae and one coccygeal vertebra (see Figure 2-2).

The medical text *Ling Ling Shu Chapter 14 - Gu Du (On the Measurement of Bones)* tells us that: "…of the top seven vertebrae, and between the first thoracic vertebra process, and in the coccygeal vertebra there are twenty one vertebrae." Also, that "The top seven vertebras" in the text are the same as the seven cervical vertebrae. These observations prove that medical scientists in ancient China counted the first seven vertebras based on vertebral segments and thoracic vertebrae, and that the segments below were counted by the spinous process. These facts confirm that the spinal bone spoken of in ancient Chinese medical texts is the spinal column (spinal vertebrae) described in modern medicine today.

Medical scientists in ancient China, as we have seen, discovered the hollows inside the spinal column. These hollows are analogous to the spinal apertures and vertebral canal studied in modern anatomy today. Both refer to the large spaces in the middle of the spine, as shown in Figure (2-3).

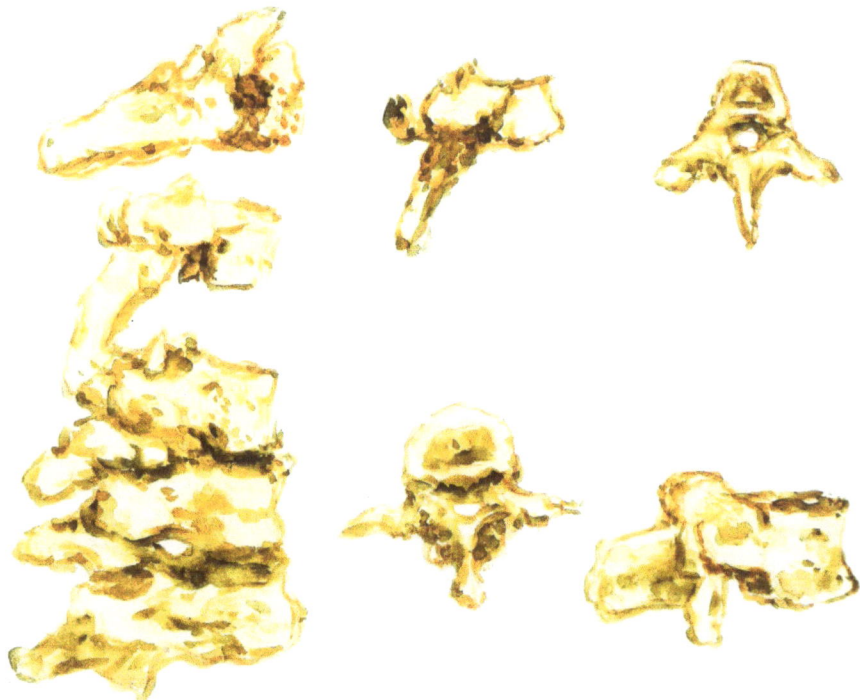

[2-2]

骨架中的脊柱，就是中国古代医学家描述的脊骨，详见图（2-2）。因不仅脊柱和脊骨都以"脊"为基础，而且数量也一致。如脊柱中有颈椎 7 节、胸椎 12 节、腰椎 5 节、骶椎 4 节、尾椎一节，详见图（2-2）。

　　《灵枢·骨度第十四》曰："……上七节和膂骨以下至尾骶二十一节"。经文中的"上七节"和颈椎 7 节一致，"从膂骨以下至尾骶二十一节"，与胸、腰、骶骨的棘突相一致。说明中国古代医学家描述的脊骨，上七节以节为准，从胸椎以下是以棘突为准。据此证明，中国古代医学家描述的脊骨，就是现代医学中描记的脊柱（脊椎）。

　　在脊骨的结构方面中国古代医学家发现了脊骨空，现代解剖学中椎孔、椎管。二者均指脊骨中间之大空（孔），详见图（2-3）。

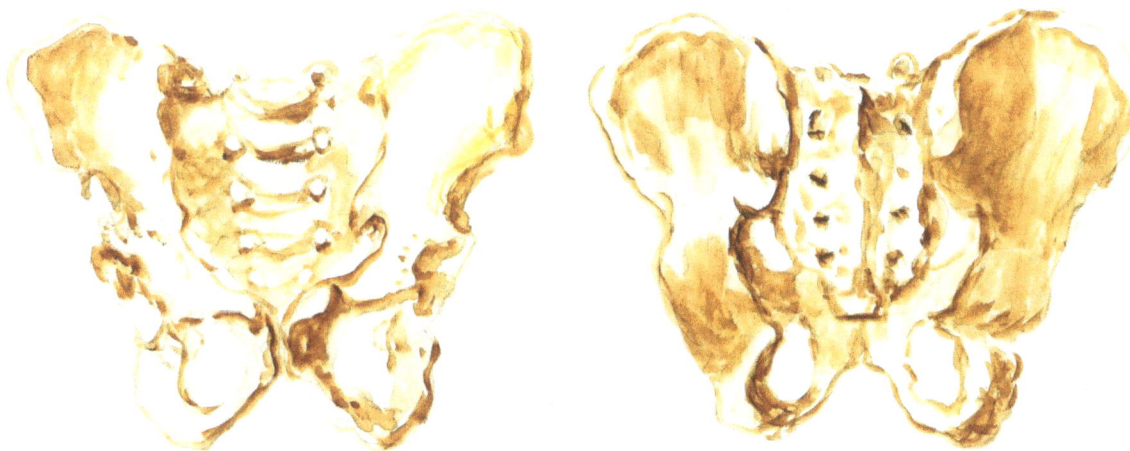

[2-3]

According to this statement, the space inside the spinal column discovered by medical scientists in ancient China is the "vertebral canal" also described in modern medicine.

If we remove the spinous process and vertebral arch at the back of the spinal column, the vertebral canal (the hollow inside the spinal column) is revealed. Starting from the first cervical vertebra (and moving down) below the sacrum, we can clearly observe the dura mater spinalis. See Figure (2-4)

This advanced level of anatomical observation was practiced by medical scientists in China over 2,000 years ago, as is evidenced by the text *Nan Jing,* Chapter 28 which says: "However, *Du mai* starts from the *Shu* point at the bottom of the spine, merges into the spinal column, goes upward to *Feng Fu,* and enters into the brain." Once the exposed dura mater spinalis and arachnoid are cut and removed, we see that the *Sui (*known to modern anatomy as bone marrow) almost fills the entire space inside the spinal column. See Figure (2-5).

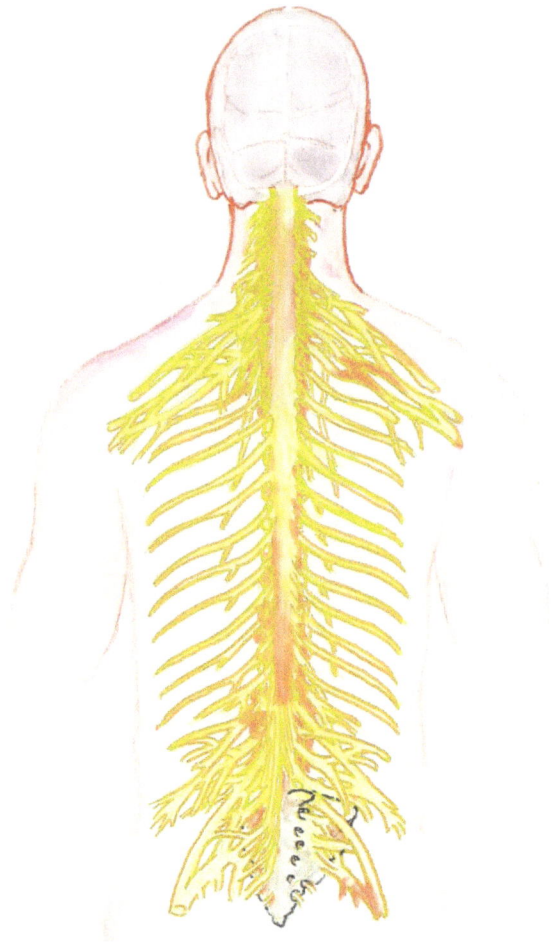

[2-4 and 5]

据此证明，中国古代医学家发现的脊骨空，就指现代医学中描述的"椎管"。

在脊柱的背面，切除棘突和椎弓，即可露出椎管（脊骨空）。从第一颈椎到骶骨之下，首先露出的是硬脊膜，见图（2-4）。

这种解剖形式，中国古代医学家早在两千年前即进行过，如《难经·二十八难》曰："然，督脉者，起于下极之俞，并于脊里，上至风府，入属于脑。"即是佐证。将暴露出的硬脊膜和蛛网膜剪开切掉，即可见到几乎充满脊骨空里的"髓"，也就是现代医学中描述的"脊髓"，详见图（2-5）。

This statement verifies that as early as 2,000 years ago Chinese doctors conducted anatomic experiments. They discovered the marrow in the hollow inside the spinal column, as well as the sea of *Jingmai*, the governor of *Jingmai,* and the pivot of *Jingmai.*

Medical scientists in ancient China discovered that *Jingmai* in the human body merge into the hollow inside the spinal column, forming the sea of *Jingmai.* They also described the way in which *Jingmai* converged and how the *Du mai* was located in the hollow inside the spinal column. They likewise knew how the *Jingmai* of the entire body are governed, and they conducted extensive medical research, achieving great advances in the field of medicine. Note, for example, in the text *Zhen Jiu Jia Yi Jing Chapter 4 - Zhen Dao*, it is said: "Crossings of *Jie*, 365 junctions. For those who know the essence, one sentence is enough; those who do not know talk pointlessly and endlessly. The so-called *Jie* are places where *Shen Qi* travels in and out, they are not skin, muscles, tendons, bones." This passage describes in detail (what we know today) as the anterolateral and posterolateral spinal tracts and neurofilaments. The front and rear roots allow the free transmissions of information in and out, and are not made of skin, muscles, tendons, or bones.

There is no record of when the above discussion was first completed. We only know that it was written many centuries ago, and that through the years scholars have argued about it but never reached a consensus. Later on, a great medical expert summarized it accurately by saying that "The so-called *Jie* are places where *Shen Qi* travels in and out; they are not skin, muscles, tendons, bones." Although these are only the words of one expert, they has been widely accepted and passed down through the centuries.

The author of *Ling Shu Chapter 1 - Nine Needles and Twelve Source Points* is not only an expert practitioner of piercing *Jingmai* to treat disease; he is also a great theorist in the research of *Jingmai*. He was familiar with and mastered an understanding of *Jingmai* in the hollows inside the spinal column, and he knew the value and significance of this finding. He boldly pioneered a method for describing *Jingmai* by starting (research in) *Jingmai* in the hollows inside the spinal column. His consequent achievements revealed the *Jingmai* to be a holistic system that deals with death and life, and that regulates the balance of the entire body. His work laid the scientific and theoretic foundations for using fine needles to pierce *Jingmai*, and for treating diseases through (energy balance and) adjustment.

据此证明，中国古代医学家，早在两千年前即进行过此类解剖，而且发现了脊骨空里髓、经脉之海、经脉之督、经脉之枢……

中国古代医学家，发现人体的经脉，汇集于脊骨空里，形成经脉之海，当然知道全身的经脉是如何汇集的。知道脊骨空里的督脉，当然知道全身经脉如何被统督的。只不过是后人在继承中，没有考虑到这些相关的内容。实际上，中国古代医学家，已经对此类问题进行过广泛而深入研究，并取得了巨大成果。《针灸甲乙经·针道第四》曰："节之交，凡365会。知其要者，一言而终；不知其要者，流散无穷。所言节者，神气之所游行出入也，非皮、肉、筋、骨也。"即是佐证。因该段经文就是对位于脊髓前外侧沟的神经根（细）丝和后外侧沟的神经根（细）丝的具体描述。因前、后根丝不仅能自由传递出入信息，而且也不是皮、肉、筋、骨。

这个成果，最早是什么年代完成的，现无据确考。只知道是很久很久以前的成果。因该论述出现的年代久远，一直争论不休，始终没有结果，后来有医学大家用，"所言节者，神气之游行出入也，非皮、肉、筋、骨也"进行准确的表述。这虽为一家之言，一直广为流传。

《九针十二原第一》的作者，不仅是微针刺经脉治病的大实践家，而且是研究经脉的大理论家。他熟悉精通中国古代医学家，对脊骨空里经脉研究的成果，他还知道这些成果的价值和意义。所以，他独辟蹊径，大胆开创了从脊骨空里经脉入手，表述人体经脉的新方法。他的这一举措，使人体的经脉，成了能决死生、调平衡的完整系统。给微针刺经脉，通过调整治病，奠定了科学理论基础。

Section 2.2 - Somatic *Jingmai*

Somatic *Jingmais* and their treatment using fine needles is of great clincial importance in Chinese acupuncture.

Because somatic *Jingmai* are pierced directly by fine needles, medical experts pay special attention to the somatic *Jingmai* and study them in depth. Due to differences of opinion, perspectives and methods vary. Here I can only summarize the research that has been done on the subject in anatomy, physiology and clinical acupuncture.

I. Research in the fields of anatomy and physiological experimentation.

Medical experts in ancient China were not only great clinical practitioners; they were astute and observant students of *Jingmai* as well. They initiated early research on *Jingmai* and made substantial achievements with their efforts. Before *Jiu Juan* there was a specialized book known as *Jingmai*. Evidence (for this) can be found in the preface of the ancient text *Zhen Jiu Jia Yi Jing* which declares that "*Jiu Juan* is the original version of the book *Jingmai*; its meaning is profound, and it is difficult to understand." *Ling Shu Chapter 1 - Nine Needles and Twelve Source Points* also pays special attention to somatic *Jingmai*. The following is a summary of related contents from this book.

(A) Crossings of Jie, 365 Hui

Zhen Jiu Jia Yi Jing Chapter 4 - Zhen Dao says: "Crossings of *Jie*, 365 hui." This sentence presents a conclusive summary of somatic *Jengmai* research. The so-called Crossings of *Jie* are the junctions of *Jie* and *Jingmai*. "*Fan 365 hui*" refers to the 365 junctions (also to *Jingmai* located deep inside the 365 acupuncture points) on the human body. These crossings are formed at multiple junctions of the *Jie* of *Jingmai,* a unique observation made via careful study of anatomy. Over the centuries, future generations did not understand this statement, and there were many contradictory and conflicting opinions concerning its true meaning. In the *Zhen Jiu Jia Yi Jing Chapter 4 - Zhen Dao*, it says: ". . . . For those who know the essence, one sentence is enough; those who do not know talk pointlessly and endlessly." *Ling Shu Chapter 1 - Nine Needles and Twelve Source Points* used this sentence to describe somatic *Jingmai*. Again, future generations did not comprehend the importance of this fact and the text was ignored for centuries.

第二节 躯肢经脉

躯肢经脉是人体经脉系统的重要组成部分。中国用微针刺躯肢治疗疾病，即是通过刺躯肢经脉治疗疾病的。因此，其在中国针刺治病中，占有重要地位。

由于用微针直接刺躯肢经脉治疗疾病，所以医学家对躯肢经脉特别关注，并进行了深入研究。因观点不同，研究的角度的方法各异。此处，仅摘述有关解剖、生理、临床针刺等研究内容。

一、通过解剖、生理试验进行研究

中国古代医学家，不仅是伟大的临床实践家，而且是杰出的经脉研究专家。对经脉的研究，不仅起源早，而且取得了丰硕成果。正因为如此，早在《九卷》之前，即有了《经脉》专著。《针灸甲乙经》序文"《九卷》是原本经脉，其义深奥，不易觉也，"即是佐证。《灵枢·九针十二原第一》也非常重视躯肢经脉，现将相关内容摘述。

（一）节之交，365 会

《针灸甲乙经·针道第四》曰："节之交，凡 365 会。"即是古代医学家，通过人体解剖，对躯肢经脉研究的结论。所谓"节之交"即是经脉之节所交。"凡 365 会。"即是经脉之节通过多次交叉，在全身形成的 365 个会（指 365 个穴位深部的经脉）。这样特殊而精准的结论，只有通过认真解剖才能得出。这句经文源于很久很久之前，因年代久远，后人不解其意，多种意见处于争论之中。《针灸甲乙经·针道第四》曰："……知其要者，一言而终；不知其要者，流散无穷。"即是佐证。《灵枢·九针十二原第一》特用该句经文表述躯肢经脉。遗憾的是后人在继承中，又因未解其意，使其一直尘封于原文之中。

(B) Shun Ni Chu Ru Zhi Hui

Ling Shu Chapter 1 - Nine Needles and Twelve Source Points pioneered a new way of describing somatic *Jingmai* as "Junctions where *Qi* flow and counter flow, exits and enters." By using "Junctions where *Qi* flow and counter flow, exits and enters" to express *Jingmai*, we know that the author of *Ling Shu Chapter 1 - Nine Needles and Twelve Source Points* was well acquainted with the fact that each somatic *Jingmai* can freely transmit information in and out (of itself). If he did not think this concept was accurate he would certainly not have included it in his book. There is no record in regard to what method was used by ancient scientists to test this theory.

Where do the somatic *Jingmai*s join? Are there flows and counter flows, entrances and exits in *Jingmai*? These questions can only be answered through a study of anatomy and physiological functions. *Jingmai*s in the hollow inside the spinal column are formed by *Jingmai*s all over the body (at the points) where they merge together. It is found that *Jingmai*s in the hollows inside the spinal column are somatic *Jingmai*s.

If we consult an anatomical textbook on the subject of neurological anatomy, we find that the nerves that pass in and out of the spinal marrow are somatic nerves. These nerves are formed by multiple junctions of the anterolateral and posterolateral spinal tracts and neurofilments. See Figures (2-6), (2-7), (2-8), (2-9), (2-10), (2-11), (2-12) and (2-13).

The somatic nerves can transmit out-going motor information and in-coming sensory information. The fact that the structural purpose of the nerve junctions and their function is to transmit information in and out is consistent with the findings of *Jingmai* as described by ancient scientists. This convergence of old theory and new proves that the somatic nerves (peripheral nerves) identified in modern medicine are the same somatic *Jingmai*s that were identified by ancient scientists.

Based on the above we know that the somatic nerves in the human body were first discovered 2,000 years ago by ancient Chinese scientists, and that this knowlege was used by Chinese doctors in their clinical practice. It was only many centuries later (during the time of the Renaissance) that the existence of the somatic nerves was discovered in the West.

（二）逆顺出入之会

《灵枢·九针十二原第一》独辟蹊径，特用"逆顺出入之会"来表述躯肢经脉。用"逆顺出入之会"来表述躯肢经脉，证明《九针十二原第一》的作者，深知每条躯肢经脉，都能自由传递出入之信息，不然也不会用其文表述的。古人最早究竟用什么方法测试的，现无据可考。

躯肢经脉是否交叉？能否逆顺出入？只有通过解剖和生理功能进一步确认。因脊骨空里的经脉。都是全身经脉汇聚而成的。查清所会脊里的经脉，即是躯肢经脉。

翻开人体解剖书，在神经解剖中，即可看到进出脊髓的是全身的躯肢神经。躯肢神经都是位于脊髓前外侧沟的神经根（细）丝和后外侧沟的神经根（细）丝，通过多次交叉而形成的。详见图（2-6），（2-7），（2-8），（2-9），（2-10），（2-11），（2-12），（2-13）。

而躯肢神经能传出运动信息和传入感觉信息。这些结构的交叉特征和逆顺出入传递信息之功能，与古人描述的躯肢经脉惊人一致。据此证明，现代医学中描述的躯肢（周围）神经，就是古代医学家描述的躯肢经脉。

由此而知，人体的躯肢神经，不是外国人、西方人先发现的。而是中国古代医学家，早在两千年前就将早已发现的躯肢神经知识，广泛应用于临床。

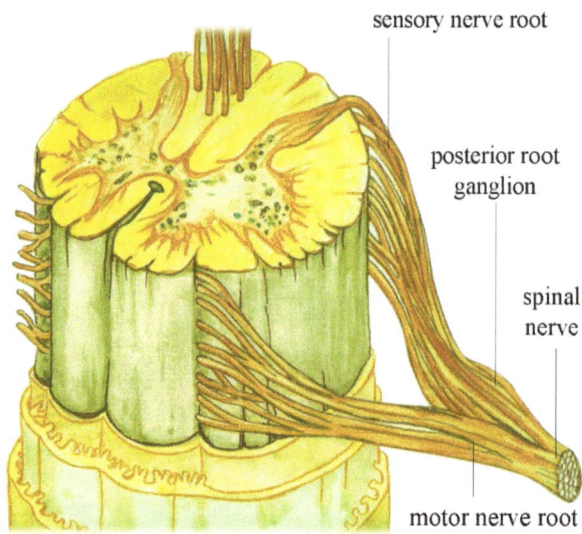

sensory nerve root

posterior root ganglion

spinal nerve

motor nerve root

[2-6]

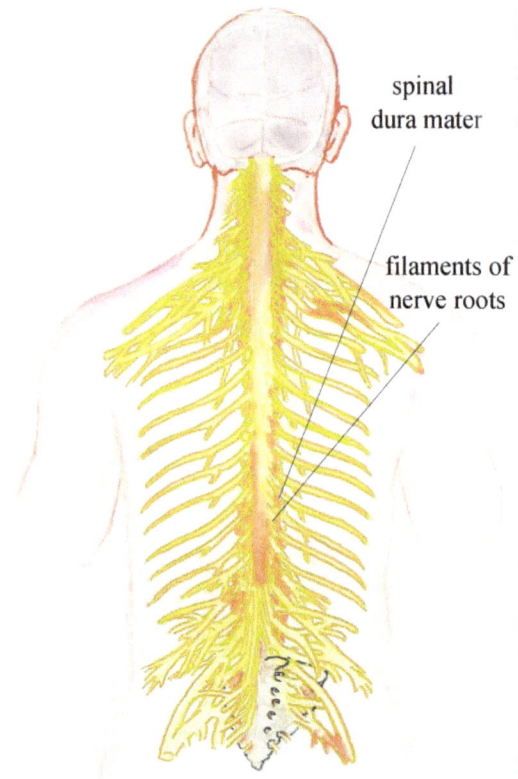

spinal dura mater

filaments of nerve roots

[2-7]

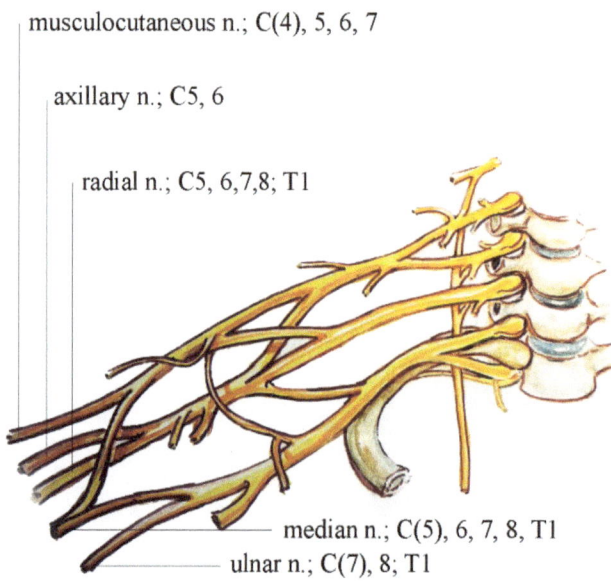

musculocutaneous n.; C(4), 5, 6, 7

axillary n.; C5, 6

radial n.; C5, 6,7,8; T1

median n.; C(5), 6, 7, 8, T1
ulnar n.; C(7), 8; T1

[2-8]

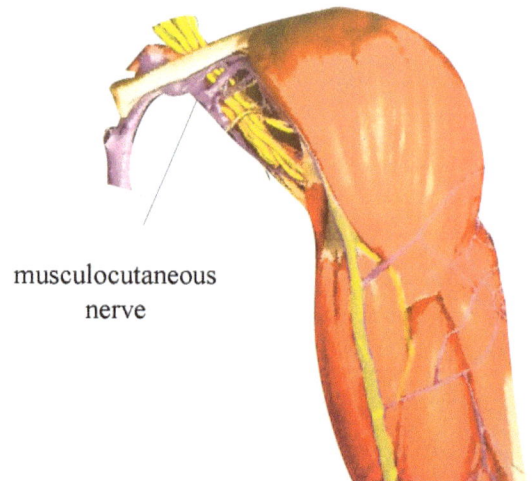

musculocutaneous nerve

[2-9]

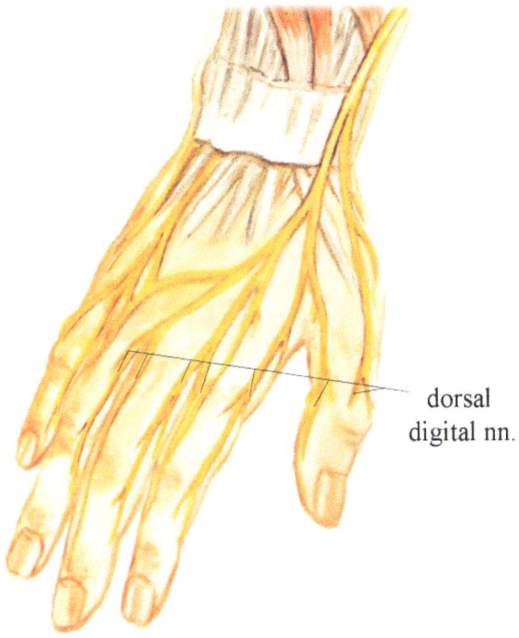

dorsal
digital nn.

[2-10]

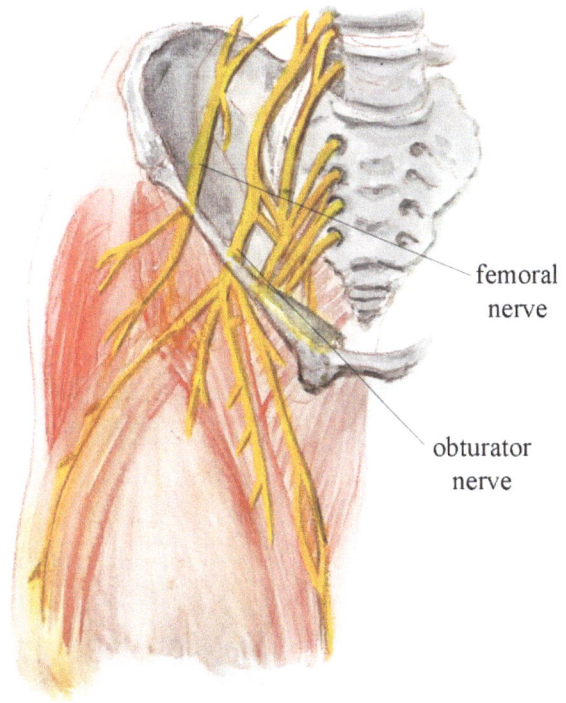

femoral
nerve

obturator
nerve

[2-11]

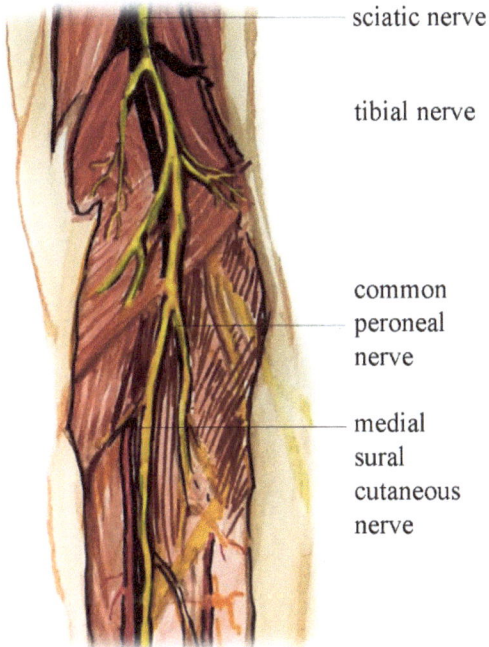

sciatic nerve

tibial nerve

common
peroneal
nerve

medial
sural
cutaneous
nerve

[2-12]

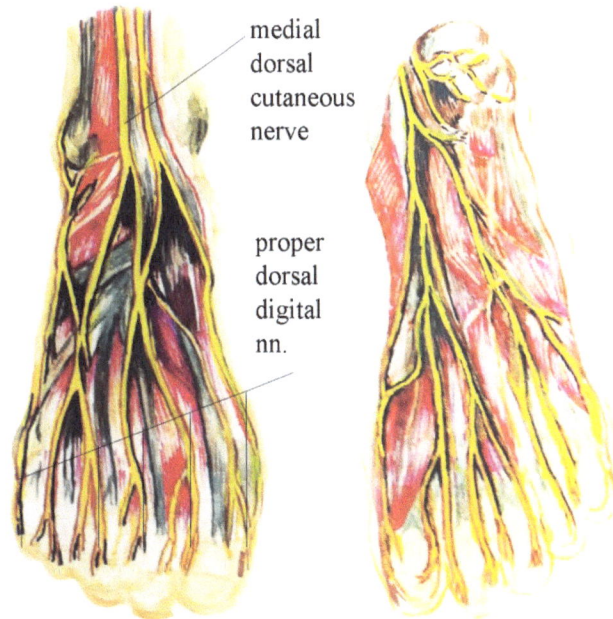

medial
dorsal
cutaneous
nerve

proper
dorsal
digital
nn.

[2-13]

Chapter III - On Using Fine Needles To Pierce *Jingmai*

Ling Shu Chapter 1 - Nine Needles and Twelve Source Points advocates the use of fine needles to pierce *Jingmai*. The sentence "I want to use fine needles to open up its *Jingmai*" provides evidence for this statement.

If we read the sentence "using fine needles to pierce *Jingmai*" in a literal way it seems like a simple statement. But in fact (through the years) it has exerted enormous scientific influence on all branches of clinical Chinese acupuncture. Although Chinese acupuncturists began to use fine needles millennia ago, many medical experts did not understand their importance in piercing the *Jingmai*. They only knew that once they pierced certain acupoints distinct healing effects could be achieved. Later, after a long period of clinical practice and in-depth research, Chinese medical experts began to make certain important observations such as the fact that "(The doctor) must pierce the *Qi* point," "pierce the *Qi* point," "pierce *Shen*," and "pierce *Ji*." Those who planned, experimented, and wrote *Ling Shu Chapter 1 - Nine Needles and Twelve Source Points* carefully summarized all this past medical experience, and used it to inform their text.

The appearance of the statement "using fine needles to pierce *Jingmai*" launched this specific practice and led to a new era of medical treatment. From that time on China's use of fine needles to pierce *Jingmai* and treat disease rapidly developed in a scientific way. Unfortunately, future generations did not understand *Ling Shu Chapter 1 - Nine Needles and Twelve Source Points* as well as they should. The result was that a complete and full understanding of the *Jingmai* was ignored and largely forgotten. This was a tragedy for the future history of Chinese medicine. Therefore, (if we are to exploit its full value) we need to truly understand the meaning of the *Ling Shu's* original text and express its ideas correctly in modern language (in order to fully profit from the wisdom of its authors). Only by so doing can we vigorously promote the ideas (of the masters who created it) and pass them on to posterity. The following interpretations are based on the meaning of the original text.

第一章 －论微针刺经脉

《灵枢·九针十二原第一》倡导用微针刺经脉，"欲以微针通其经脉"即是佐证。

"微针刺经脉"，从字面上看很简单。实际上，它对中国针刺治病，有非常重要的科学价值。因为在很久很久以前，中国虽然就应用微针刺经脉治病了。但是，在那个时段，很多医学家并不知道被刺的是经脉，只知道在穴位中将微针刺在某特定物上，即能获得明显疗效。后来，经过长期临床实践和深入研究，积累了很多经验，"必中气穴"、"中气穴"、"刺神"、"刺机"……就是部分佐证。《九针十二原第一》的决策者、策划者、试验者、实践者，认真总结了过去的相关经验，结合对人体进行解剖、针刺试验等，证明了过去所记述的那些经验，即是微针刺经脉的经验，才特意提出"微针通其经脉"的。

微针刺经脉的出现，开创了微针刺经脉治病的先河，使针刺治病垮入了科学治病的新时代。此后，中国的微针刺经脉治病，本应沿着科学轨迹，快速向前发展。但遗憾的是，因后人没有读懂《九针十二原第一》，逼使微针刺经脉的技术，一直尘封在原文中。这是中国微针刺经脉技术史上一大悲剧。令人揪心。据此，我们不仅要真正读懂原文，并且要用现代语言正确表述。只有这样，才能大力弘扬、不断传承。现据原文之意进行论述。

Section 3.1 - Fine Needles

By using fine needles to treat disease, and by observing the fact that patients tended to improve when treated this way, Chinese doctors thousands of years ago invented the art of fine needle acupuncture. Through the years fine needles were continuously improved in terms of their quality, width, and length. There is, however, no documented evidence regarding when fine needles actually first appeared, though it is estimated that they were in wide use as early as 3,500 years ago. *Ling Shu Chapter 1 - Nine Needles and Twelve Source Points* says: "*The Great Essentials* says: 'Slow then rapid is excess. Rapid then slow is deficiency.'" This statement offers evidence that fine needle acupuncture was in clinical use at a very early date.

Ling Shu Chapter 1 - Nine Needles and Twelve Source Points emphatically encourages the use of fine needles to treat disease, giving fine needle acupuncture a special purpose and mission. Since the time of its writing fine needles were widely used for piercing *Jingmai* to treat diseases.

Medical scientists in ancient China invented fine needles thousands of years ago and used them to pierce the *Jingmais* to treat diseases, thus proving the value of this treatment many times over. These early practitioners deserve to be congratulated!

The purpose of discussing fine needles is to understand (their use, function, and value) correctly. In the future, acupuncture *Jingmais* for treating disease will continue to use fine needles exclusively.

Section 3.2 - Holding Needles

The way to hold a needle is an important aspect of acupuncture *Jingmais*. The Jingmais can *only* be stimulated correctly if practitioners grip the needle in the proper way.

Ling Shu Chapter 1 - Nine Needles and Twelve Source Points says: "As for the way to hold a needle, holding it in a firm way is precious." The statement "holding it in a firm way is precious" does not imply that the firmer one grips a needle the better. It is saying that it is good to hold the needle firmly when piercing the body and *Jingmai,* but not to hold it *too* firmly. In truth, it is extremely difficult to explain how to master one's grip on a needle. One can only learn this art thoroughly through (long years of) clinical experience.

第一节 – 微针

"微针"是中国医学专家，在数千年前，通过针刺治病的临床实践，逐步改进、完善而形成的。其出现的最早年代，现无据可考。但据有关资料推测，早在3500 年前，已经被广泛应用，并积累了丰富经验。《灵枢·九针十二原第一》曰："《大要》曰：'徐而疾则实，疾而徐则虚'"，即是描述用微针刺经脉治疗疾病的佐证。后来，在临床实践中，对微针的质量、粗细、长度，不断进行改进。

《灵枢·九针十二原第一》特别倡导，用微针刺经脉治病。这一举措，使微针有了特殊用途和使命。从那时起，微针就一直担当起刺经脉治病的重任。

中国古代医学家发明了"微针"，并应用其刺经脉治病，持续数千年不衰。证明"微针"价值非凡、意义重大，可喜可贺！

谈"微针"、论"微针"， 目的是为了正确认识"微针"，认真对待"微针"。因在今后针刺经脉治病的年月里，仍然只能用"微针"。

第二节　持针

持针是针刺经脉的一个重要环节，因为只有正确持针，才能刺中经脉。

《灵枢·九针十二原第一》曰："持针之道，坚者为宝"。经文之意是"紧握针"。我认为应正确理解"坚者为宝"之意。它不是握的越紧越好，而是只要握住针能刺入体内和经脉，即为合适度，过度用力大可不必。当然要掌控好持握针的力量，目前很难用量化概念说清楚。只有通过针刺治病的临床实践，不断积累经验，才能持握适度，运用自如。

Section 3.3 - Pierce into the Skin

Using a fine needle to pierce the skin is the first step in applying *Jingmai* acupuncture. As a result, it is important (for the doctor) to practice piercing in an effective manner. There are two issues to be aware of in this regard. First, if we are to pierce the *Jingmai* accurately we must needle the point in the proper way. Second, we must pierce through the skin quickly in order to reduce the patient's pain.

Section 3.4 - The Direction of Piercing

When it comes to the direction of needling, *Ling Shu Chapter 1 - Nine Needles and Twelve Source Points* provides two descriptions:

I. Pierce perpendicularly

First, the sentence "*Zheng zhi zhi ci, wu zhen zuo you*" tells us to pierce perpendicularly and to not (incline the) needle to the left or right.

II. The direction that triggers the "arrival of *Qi*" is the correct direction

The direction that triggers the "arrival of *Qi*" is the correct direction. If *Qi* does not arrive the technique is incorrect. "When *Qi* goes away, it is called counter flow (*Ni*); when it arrives, it is called flow (*Shun*). When counter flow and flow are grasped, positive (healing) actions can be taken without (doubts or) questions" tells us that if the "arrival of *Qi*" occurs when pushing in a needle this means the direction of the needle is correct (a condition termed "*Shun*"). On the other hand, a direction that makes the "arrival of *Qi*" weak or causes it to dissipate is the wrong direction (which is termed "*Ni*"). As long as you know the *Shun* and *Ni*, pierce boldly with no more questions.

In clinical practice both the above methods are useful. We should use them flexibly according to the locations of the acupuncture point and the specific requirements of a given treatment. All in all, the number one choice of needle direction is the direction that best triggers the "arrival of *Qi*."

第三节 - 刺入皮肤

将微针刺入皮肤，是针刺经脉的第一步，也是必由之路。所以，刺皮关一定要过好。其中有两个问题需要注意。首先是刺入点要相对准确，因其直接关系到刺中经脉的准确率。其次是要快速刺入皮肤，因快速刺入能大大减轻病人的痛感。

第四节 - 刺入方向

关于针刺入的方向，在《灵枢·九针十二原第一》中有两种描述：

一、垂直刺入

"正指直刺，无针左右"，即是垂直刺入的佐证。

二、能出现"气至"的方向，则为正确刺入方向

能出现"气至"的方向，则为正确刺入方向，反之，则不然。"往者为逆，来者为顺；明知逆顺，正行无问" 即是在将针往进推时，如能出现"气至"者，则为正确方向，简称"顺"。相反，如果使"气至"消退或消失的方向，为不正确方向，简称"逆"。只要知道了"逆"、"顺"之意，就大胆去刺，再不要问了。

在临床实践中，两种方法都有用。应据穴位所在部位和针刺治疗的特殊要求灵活掌握。总之，应以能出现"气至"为首选的针刺方向。

Section 3.5 - Pierce the *Jingmais*

Piercing *Jingmais* is the core technique that determines the success or failure of a treatment. Therefore, one must be familiar with this technique and practice it carefully. For better understanding, I will discuss it in three aspects.

I. Why should we pierce the *Jingmai*?

Ling Shu Chapter 1 - Nine Needles and Twelve Source Points considers piercing *Jingmai* to be the key to successful acupuncture treatment. The reason why acupuncture has achieved so much success over thousands of years is that it concentrates on piercing the *Jingmai*. Thus, we must seek to pierce the *Jingmai*. Here are some examples.

"A poor doctor only looks for the physical location of an acupoint, while a superior doctor seeks the spirit (*Shen*)." The "spirit" mentioned here is wondrous; it is "like a distinguished guest entering our door". This passage means that the inferior doctor knows only how to needle the physical location of the acupuncture points, while a superior doctor knows (how to find) the *Shen* in a point. That is, a superior doctor knows how to pierce the *Shen* in the *Jingmai* to treat disease. *Shen* is therefore a miraculous force. It is like an honorable guest who we welcome inside the *Jingmai*.

"A poor doctor only knows how to look for the physical joints (*Guan*) while the superior doctor knows how to find *Ji* – gate mechanismin in the point. The movement of *Qi* never exceeds its space. When we observe it from the outside *Qi* activity appears tranquil in the space it occupies. It appears to have only a slight movement. Its coming cannot be met and its going cannot be followed or grasped. Those who understand the gate mechanism are able to pierce the points precisely without missing a hair's breadth. Those who do not understand gate mechanism will miss the timing of *Qi*. Piercing points in a random way is useless. Knowing where *Qi* is coming from and where it is going and timing of *Qi* to get the best result is important. This phenomenon is really wondrous. The poor doctor remains in the dark (about it), while the superior doctor knows all these (important facts). "

第五节 – 刺经脉

刺经脉是核心技术，成败在此一举。所以，必须熟悉掌握，认真操作。为了便于理解，分三点进行描述。

一、为什么要刺经脉？

《九针十二原第一》认为，刺经脉是针刺治病的关键。几千年来，中国针刺治病能取得较好疗效，就是因为刺中经脉。所以，现在必须要求刺中经脉。为了证明上述论点，特举一些实例。

"粗守形，上守神；神乎神，客在门"。该段经文之意即是说，低劣的医生，只知道针刺穴位治病。而高明的医生，即知道在穴位中刺神治病。神非常神奇，就像贵客位于穴位之中。这里所讲的"神"，实指"经脉"。

逢，其往不可追。知机之道，不可挂以发；不知机道，叩之不发。知其往来，要与之期。粗之暗乎，妙哉！工独有之。"

This passage means that the inferior doctor only knows how to apply needles to the physical points when treating disease, while the superior doctor knows how to find and pierce the *Ji* in these locations. Through anatomical and physiological experiment (including observation), it has been found that the movement of *Ji* never exceeds its space. *Ji* activity appears tranquil when we look at it from the outside. It only shows slight movement. But the activities going on within *Ji* are swift and delicate, transmitting information in and out. This phenomenon is difficult to detect with the naked eye. Those doctors who understand the essence of *Ji* will pierce it precisely; those who do not understand the essence of *Ji* will find (the *Ji* in the point) difficult to locate and pierce. By knowing the coming and going of *Ji* one can achieve the anticipated (healing) goal. This is a miraculous fact an inferior doctor cannot see (into the essence of needling practice); only a superior doctor knows (what to do).

II. How do we decide whether the *Jingmai* is pierced?

Somatic *Jingmais* are located deep in the body. We cannot see them, nor can we see whether or not the needle has pierced them accurately. Ancient Chinese medical experts described the experience and insights they attained through clinical practice and the needling of the *Jingmai*. These are summarized as follows:

1. When we push the needle into the acupuncture point, if the resistance at the tip of the needle suddenly grows stronger this pressure means that the *Jingmai* is pierced. Otherwise the *Jingmai* is not pierced. (The important point is to sense when the resistance grows stronger)

Ling Shu Chapter 1 - Nine Needles and Twelve Source Points says: "*The Great Essentials* says: 'Slow then rapid is excess. Rapid then slow is deficiency.'" The meaning of this statement is that when we push a needle into an acupuncture point and the resistance at the tip of the needle suddenly becomes strong this means it is "firm" and that the needle has successfully pierced the *Jingmai*. On the other hand, if there is little or no resistance at the tip of the needle this indicates that the needle is still in a state of "emptiness." This condition of emptiness is called "*Xu*" and means that the *Jingmai* is not pierced. This feeling in the needle is very unique. It manifests as a sudden increase of resistance rather than the (even) resistance encountered as the needle slides in. This feeling, referred to as "*wan chen*," often occurs when the needle reaches the tendons and bones. When we experience this sensation we should withdraw the needle a small amount, change direction, and pierce again. *The Great Essentials* is an ancient text and its words prove that the above information was understood and put into practice long ago.

该段经文之意即是说，低劣的医生只知道针刺穴位治病，而高明的医生则知道在穴位中刺"机"治病。通过解剖和生理试验（含观察）发现，"机"仅在其空间活动。从表面上看"机"很宁静，仅有轻微之动，其内部活动快速灵敏，传递出入信息，在此过程主观常常不易觉察。知道"机"的要害，就很容易刺中。不知道"机"的要害，即很难刺中。知道"机"的来龙去脉，就能达到预期目的。低劣的医生什么也看不见，真奇妙！只有高明的医生才知道这一切。

二、怎样才算刺中经脉？

躯肢经脉位于人体表的深部，用眼睛看不见，当然更看不到针是否刺中经脉。但是，中国古代医学家，通过临床实践，早已总结出很多刺中经脉的经验和感悟。现摘述于后：

1、在穴位中将针往进刺时，如针尖处突然阻力变大，即可视其刺中经脉。反之，则不然。（这里要注意，关键是变大。）

《灵枢·九针十二原第一》曰："《大要》曰：'徐而疾则实，疾而徐则虚'"。该段经文之意即是说，在穴位中将针微往进推，突然针尖处阻力变大，为"实"。即表示针已刺中经脉。反之，如果针往进推的比较快，针尖处出现阻力很小或完全没有阻力，即表示针尖仍在"虚"处，简称"虚"，即证明没有刺中经脉。这种感觉很特别，必须是突然变成的阻力。而不是将针往进推时，遇到的阻力，这种情况往往是针尖刺在肌腱、骨骼等，这种阻力古代医学家称"宛陈"，这时应将针往后推，改变方向再刺。因《大要》是上古篇名，证明这一经验来源于很久以前。

2. Once the "arrival of *Qi* (*De Qi*) occurs, it proves that the *Jingmai* is pierced."

Ling Shu Chapter 1 - Nine Needles and Twelve Source Points says: "(if you) pierce and *Qi* does not arrive, do not ask how many times (you have pieced); (if you) pierce and *Qi* arrives, remove the needle and (perform) no more piercing." The meaning of this passage is that if the "arrival of *Qi*" does not occur when piercing, keep piercing and do not ask how many times (you must continue) to pierce. Once the "arrival of *Qi*" occurs remove the needle and stop piercing.

The essence of this passage is that we must seek to trigger *Qi Zhi* (the arrival of *Qi*) when practicing acupuncture *Ling Shu Chapter 1 - Nine Needles and Twelve Source Points* uses this passage to show that *Qi Zhi* signals the fact that *Jingmai* has been pierced. This description is of great significance. The understanding of acupuncture advanced considerably due to the practice of *Qi Zhi* and it remains very valuable (up to today).

The occurrence of *Qi Zhi* is a very important sign. It signifies that *Jingmai* has been pierced, and it foretells that relatively good (healing) results can now be expected. *Ling Shu Chapter 1 - Nine Needles and Twelve Source Points* tells us that: "The essence of needling is that once *Qi* arrives there is a (healing) response. This response appears quickly in the way that a sudden wind blows away the clouds and the sky becomes clear and blue. This is the complete *Tao* of needling. This is the evidence."

III. Piercing the *Jingmai* should be done in a moderate way

Ling Shu Chapter 1 - Nine Needles and Twelve Yuan-Source Points suggests that acupuncturists should not only pierce *Jingmai*, but that they should practice needling with extreme moderation. Medical experts in ancient China accumulated a great deal of clinical experience when practicing acupuncture. *Ling Shu Chapter 1 - Nine Needles and Twelve Yuan-Source Points* affirms (the validity) of these experiences and the need for stimulating the *Jingmai* in a moderate way.

2. 一旦出现"气至"（得气），即证明已刺中经脉。

《灵枢·九针十二原第一》曰："刺之而气不至，无问其数；刺之而气至，乃去之，无复针。"经文之意即是，在针刺的时候，只要不出现"气至"，就不要问刺多少次一直刺。在针刺时，一旦出现"气至"，就将针取掉，不要再刺了。

该段经文的核心内容是，针刺必须出现"气至"。而《九针十二原第一》用该段经文表述，"气至"出现即标志着刺中经脉。这种表述意义深远，认识有了质的飞跃，即从针刺出现"气至"的经验，上升到针刺经脉的高度，难能可贵。

"气至"现象，非常重要。因其出现不仅能代表刺中经脉，而且也预示能出现较好疗效。《九针十二原第一》曰："刺之要，气至而有效；效之信，若风之吹云，明乎若见苍天，刺之道毕矣。"即是佐证。

三、刺经脉要讲究适度

《九针十二原第一》不仅要求刺中经脉，而且还要达到最佳适度。因中国古代医学家，在针刺治病的实践中，早就积累了丰富经验《九针十二原第一》只是认可这类经验，为刺中经脉适度的经验。

Ling Shu Chapter 1 - Nine Needles and Twelve Yuan-Source Points says: "For those who practice acupuncture, (treat) deficiency by filling, excess by draining, chronic stagnation by eliminating and over abundance of evil *Qi* by withdrawing." This passage means that for those who practice acupuncture, if there is emptiness one should fill it. If there is fullness one should drain it. When the needle encounters "*wan chen*" (a situation where the tip of the needle reaches the tendons and bones), one should remove the needle. If the patient experiences severe shivering, numbness, or pain when the needle pierces the *Jingmai* (which is called "*Xie Shen*" accoding to ancient experts), one should weaken it. The original purpose of this text is to describe the reactions that can occur during acupuncture treatment and the specific solutions for these reactions. *Ling Shu Chapter 1 - Nine Needles and Twelve Yuan-Source Points* considers that these methods can be used to adjust the intensity of piercing *Jingmai,* and to achieve optimal and appropriate treatment. "Drain is called *Ying* and tonify is called 'follow.'" This is a classical statement that refers to adjusting the intensity of *Qi Zhi.*

To sum up, *Ling Shu Chapter 1 - Nine Needles and Twelve Yuan-Source Points* suggests that one should try to acupuncture *Jingmai* and that one should be moderate (in so doing). Generally speaking, when using acupuncturing *Jingmai* it should be obvious when *Qi Zhi* (arrival of *Qi*) occurs, but the sensation of its arrival should not be too strong. The best and most appropriate degree of *Qi Zhi* is when it is bearable for the patient. That said, to practice this method really well is not an easy task. One can only do so by reflecting continuously and by taking note of one's experiences in clinical practice. According to *Nine Needles and Twelve Source Points*, care must be taken in moderation when needling the *Jingmai.* In general, moderate "arrival of *Qi*" is ideal. Many acupuncturists attempt to trigger obvious "arrival of *Qi*" during treatment, but this arrival should not be so strong that the patient cannot tolerate it. (All in all, therefore) the above are mere words, but what really needs to be done in these circumstances is not an easy thing (to explain) or do. Only by intense clinical practice and repeated summary (and research) can the practice of *Jingmai* needling be mastered.

To sum up, the technique of using fine needles to acupuncture *Jingmai* as advocated and described by *Nine Needles and Twelve Source Points* is extremely important (in the practice of medicine). It has enormous scientific value and has made enormous contributions to Chinese acupuncture. We must understand this method correctly, take it seriously, promote it vigorously, and pass it on devotedly to future generations.

《九针十二原第一》曰："凡用针者，虚则实之，满则泄之，宛陈则除之，邪胜则虚之。"该段经文之意即是，凡用针刺者，在较虚时则让其实一些；如果太满了，就应往外泄；遇到宛陈（针尖刺到肌腱、骨骼等）则应排除；针刺时出现的抽、麻、痛太明显（古人称邪胜）则应让其变的弱一些。从经文原意，只是表述在针刺时这些特殊感受及具体处理方法。而《九针十二原第一》则认为，这类感悟和处理方法，即是调整刺中经脉的程度，使其达到最佳适度的感悟和方法。"泻曰迎之，补曰随之"，即是描述调控"气至"强度的经典说法。

总之，《九针十二原第一》要求刺中经脉必须注意适度。一般来说，在针刺经脉时，既要求出现较明显的"气至"，又不能太过强，以病人能忍受为最佳适度。话是这样说的，但真正要做好，就不是一件容易的事。只有在临床实践中，不断体会，反复总结，才能越做越好。

综上所述可知，《九针十二原第一》所倡导和描述的"微针刺经脉"技术，有非常重要的科学价值。对中国的微针刺经脉治病有重大贡献。我们必须正确认识，认真对待，大力弘扬，坚决传承。

Afterword

"Acupuncture somatic *Jingmai* to treat diseases" is the most distinctive healing feature of Chinese acupuncture.

The initiation of "Acupuncture somatic *Jingmai* to treat diseases" is a great pioneering work and has contributed significant research to Chinese medicine. It is the invention of Chinese medical experts, but it is also the achievement of world medical science.

Jiao Shun Fa
March 18, 2007

"Unique healing effect" offers a great competitive advantage in the Chinese art of acupuncture *Jingmai* for treating diseases.

Acupuncture *Jingmai* as invented by Chinese doctors treats various ailments all over the body and exerts unique healing effects on certain dieseases. As far as we know, no other medical treatment method can match (or surpass) it.

Jiao Shun Fa
March 18, 2007

As summarized and advocated by the ancient text *Ling Shu Chapter 1 - Nine Needles and Twelve Yuan-Source Points*, using fine needles to acupuncture *Jingmai* marks the maturity and high point of Chinese acupuncture's attempts to treat disease. It is the most significant research method that has ever evolved from Chinese acupuncture treatment.

Jiao Shun Fa
March 18, 2007

后记

"针刺躯肢经脉治病"是中国针刺治病的最大特色。

创用"针刺躯肢经脉治病",是中国医学的伟大创举和重大科研成果。它是中国医学家的发明,也是世界医学的成就。

焦顺发

2007 年 3 月 18 日

"独特疗效"是中国针刺经脉治病的最大优势。

中国发明的针刺经脉治病,能治疗全身多种疾病,其中对某些疾病有独特疗效。到目前为止,其它治病方法皆不可替代。

焦顺发

2007 年 3 月 18 日

《灵枢·九针十二原第一》,总结和倡导的微针刺经脉治病,是中国针刺治病真正的成熟和崛起,是中国针刺治病最大的科研成果

焦顺发

2007 年 3 月 18 日

The method of using fine needles to acupuncture *Jingmai* and treat disease, as pioneered and advocated by the ancient text *Ling Shu Chapter 1 - Nine Needles and Twelve Yuan-Source Points* offers us a miraculous technique that is based on sound scientific theory and unique healing effects. As long as we understand this method correctly and consider it in a serious light, it will be like a towering tree (for all medical practitioners to see), standing tall in the forest of world medical science.

Jiao Shun Fa
March 18, 2007

Statements offered in the ancient text *Ling Shu Chapter 1 - Nine Needles and Twelve Yuan-Source Points* represent the core of *Ling Shu* and the essence of Chinese acupuncture treatment. It has great scientific value and practical significance. We must promote it vigorously and pass it on (to future generations) seriously.

Jiao Shun Fa
March 18, 2007

In short, as I read the *Nine Needles and Twelve Yuan-Source Points* I was filled with so much excitement, admiration, and inspiration that I cannot express my true esteem in ordinary words.

Jiao Shun Fa
March 18, 2007

《灵枢·九针十二原第一》创立和倡导的，"微针刺经脉治病"，是理论科学、疗效独特的绝妙方法。只要我们能正确认识、认真对待，它就能像参天大树一样，屹立在世界医林之中。

焦顺发
2007 年 3 月 18 日

《九针十二原第一》是《灵枢》的核心和中国针刺治病的精华，有重要科学价值和现实意义。我们必须大力弘扬、认真传承。

焦顺发
2007 年 3 月 18 日

总之，读《九针十二原第一》，激情四溢，感慨万千，悟叹多多，难于言表……

焦顺发
2007 年 3 月 18 日

針道通古今

焦順發

"The Dao of Acupuncture Throughout The Past And Present"
Calligraphy by Dr. Jiao

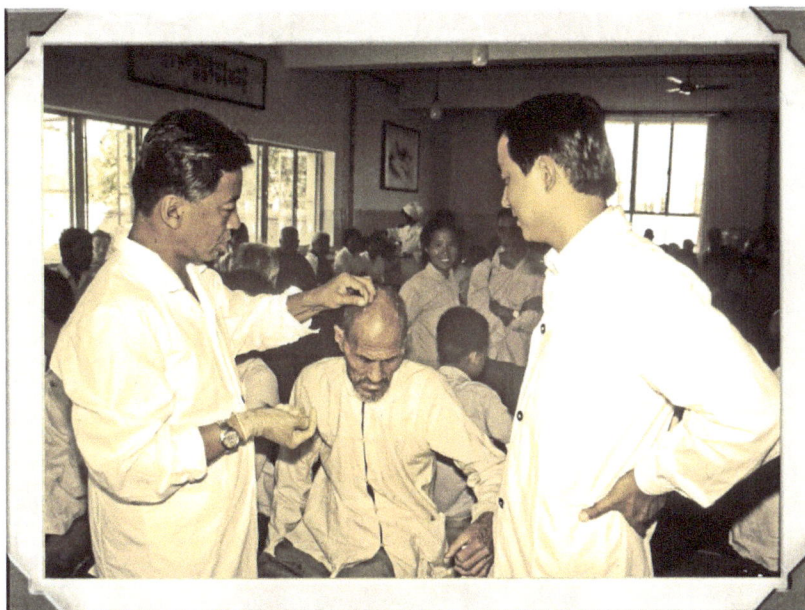
Dr. Jiao performing head acupuncture while Dr. Chan observes.

Dr. Tsoi Nam Chan has been a special friend and student of mine for almost 40 years. He is a gifted practitioner of the healing arts, as well as a master artist and calligrapher in the classical Chinese tradition. He is able to see and understand the connection between all aspects of life, which is evident in both his paintings and his approach to medicine. For Dr. Chan, treatment is more than just inserting needles; it is an all-encompassing art form that includes elements of *Qi Gong*, *Tai Qi*, *Feng Shui*, calligraphy, poetry, science, and philosophy.

Dr. Chan, moreover, is well versed in Western therapeutics as well as traditional Chinese medicine, and comfortably bridges the gap between ancient and modern forms of healing. His command of the English language plays an important part in his ability to translate deeply esoteric Chinese medical theories into clear English. For almost 30 years, his office located in New York City next to the United Nations has been filled with a healing spirit, as well as many interesting works of art. His patients comprised of people from all walks of life including foreign dignitaries, artists, celebrities and CEO's of Fortune Five Hundred companies.

There are not many people with whom I am able to discuss the content of my teachings. Dr. Chan is one of them. He truly comprehends the depth and nature of these principles, and is able to offer critical feedback and valuable advice. I am fortunate to know him as a friend, a colleague with whom I can discuss and share ideas, and as an intermediary through whom I can express important new interpretations of ancient wisdom in a way that is practical, logical and understandable. In addition to his help in translating, I would like to thank him for his designs and illustrations throughout this book.   Dr. Jiao Shun Fa